Dr. Mark Sexton N.D. PhD

SIMPLY...

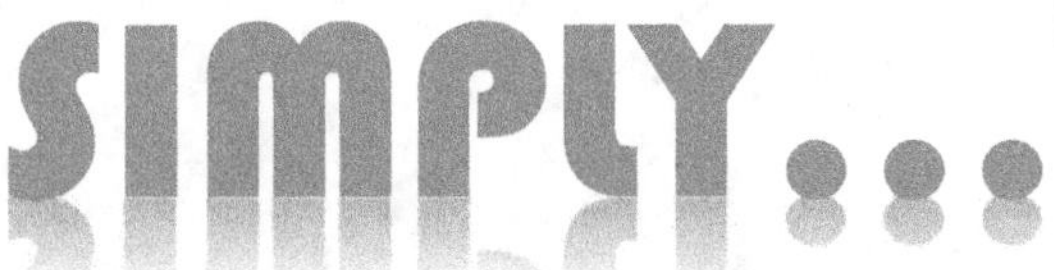

"WELL"

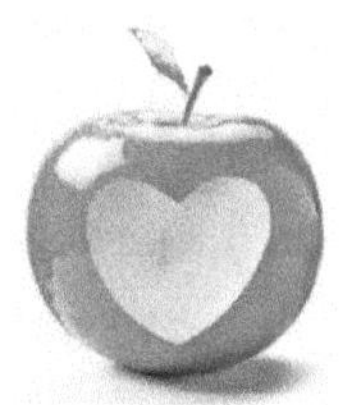

Effective Alternative Therapies

Table of Contents

Introduction

Are you running out of gas mid-day? Forgetting where you were going in the middle of a sentence? Can't knock off those extra pounds, no matter what you've slugged them with? Got re-occurring allergies or illnesses you just can't seem to shake and you're on so many meds you want to choke? If you suffer from high blood pressure, arthritis, gout, diabetes, allergies, acid reflux, restless leg syndrome, cancer or any other ailment, this book's for you.

Want more energy, get rid of those aches, pains and gnarly joints, lose the cloudy-brain syndrome? Want to get off the meds and take back charge of your life? Want to regain your youth and add quality years to your life? Rid yourself of incurable or degenerative disease while preventing them from ever haunting you again? Then, stay with me here, 'cause you're about to learn it all.

I'm Doctor Mark. Now….

Let's

Get

You

Well!

FOREWARD

The reason in writing this book is to give you the knowledge and formulas I have discovered and acquired over the last forty-four years of my career as a Naturopathic Doctor, for you to build a healthy, everlasting, non-destructible body that will enjoy perfect health for many years to come. And the best thing is, it doesn't matter how young or old you are when you start. What matters is, you start.

"Old Age" is nothing more than a space in the events of your life story. What it isn't, is an excuse to stop living, to stop caring, to feel worthless and sorry for yourself, to let everything go, to stop exercising, to become lazy and lying around just waiting for the Ol' Sweet Chariot to swing low and miss you, because you didn't even have the energy to stand up and get on board as it went by.

It's time to send that sucker on down the road and stand up and say, "I'm just beginning to live!" Don't EVER let anyone tell you, "That's just a sign of old age." That person is suffering from his or her own lack of knowledge. Well, guess what, after reading this book, you will be able to help that person, because you WILL have the knowledge.

Your body is made to regenerate itself. When you hit seventy and eighty years of age, you've just reached the expiration date of your factory warranty. Now, it's time to renew that ol' dog and get a new extended warranty plan. So called "Old Age" symptoms are just a sign of toxic accumulations in your tissues. It's a sign from your body saying, "Help me, I'm polluted. My parts are sticking, and I can't move through all this sludge." Clean 'em out and get back out there and live!

From this day forward, we're going to remove the term "Old Age" from our vocabulary and replace it with the new term "Kiddagain." Doesn't that have a much more positive feel? And it completely takes away any dogma or labeling about age-related ailments or stupid rules placed upon a person due to their age.

Right about now, you might be thinking, "This guy's crazy!"

But the world, in all its complexity, still remains, simple. We just see us as being "superior beings." So, it must be complex if we don't understand it. But the truth is, we just don't see it. It's so simple we overlook the understanding of it. Genius is no more than seeing complexity in a simplistic but structured form or "formula."

Ever talk to a computer geek that throws out computer jargon like you are supposed to know what they're talking about and every sentence out of their mouth is interrupted by, "Excuse me, but I don't have a clue what you just said?" That's because they have figured it out to a state of simplicity and to them, everyone should be able to understand the simplicity of computers. Health is not hard and you're not stupid. You just lack the knowledge. This is what I want to show you and teach you here, "The simplicity of getting and keeping yourself well."

When all is said and done and you have finished this book, you will know how to get yourself well and keep yourself well. It's all a matter of removing the garbage and rebuilding the barn. The best thing about it all; it doesn't take nearly as long to repair the damage as it took to do the damage. We're talking months and sometimes only weeks, instead of years. You can return that tired, rundown rig back to that natural state of "perfection."

At our health retreat, Castle in the Clouds, I see many patients a week and am presented many challenges and asked numerous questions. As we go along, I will address the majority of those, most frequently asked questions and problems.

I'm going to talk to you just as I do any of my patients, like we're talking face-to-face.

You were put on this earthly journey with everything in your backpack you need to survive. The one and only thing lacking is the knowledge of what and how to use some of it. So, if you're ready to continue on that journey, let's get goin'!

CHAPTER 1
ELECTRIC-ECLECTIC YOU

Now, before we go any further, we need to briefly discuss and understand a few things. Contrary to what the reflection in the mirror tells you, you are not one giant organism. In fact, you aren't even solid. Every single molecule that makes up your entire being, is separated by what is called "interstitial spaces." Each cell is made up of 100 trillion atoms and each atom is 99.9999% empty space. Now, how solid are you?

You are a cellular community or a "cell hotel" comprised of over 75 trillion individual cells, (That's about 7 quadrillion 500 trillion atoms that just make up your cells), each with their own individual jobs and set of rules programmed through DNA and each also containing their own set of systems, i.e. brain, digestive, respiratory, endocrine, etc. In other words, each individual, teeny-tiny cell has all the physiological systems as the big body has. Which is fascinating in itself, and we will be getting into that later.

I'm getting really excited. We are going to have so much fun and I have so many interesting things to share with you.

Every cell is its own power generating plant.
Did you know: the membrane of each one of these cells is capable of generating .07V (volts) of electricity.

If each cell is producing this amount of energy, that's a total of 4 trillion plus volts for the entire 75 trillion cells. That is a measurement of a cell in normal activity. Think if we were to measure and add up the voltage sum of all the cells during physical activity; it can reach output voltages of 50 trillion plus volts. Now, that's a lot of energy. And you say you're getting old? Nonsense. Your generator just needs overhauled.

You have heard a person referred to as having an "electric personality." Well, you're about to see, you and all other humans have electric personalities.

You <u>are</u> electric. Every cell or molecule that moves or rubs against another molecule, whether through blood flow, muscle movement, breathing, digestion or whatever, generates electricity. In fact, everything that happens inside your body is making electricity. You are an electric generating power plant. Isn't that exciting?

WHAT MAKES YOU DEAD?

"I'm not dead!" Okay, but if you were…

Did you know, if you were to fall over dead right now, right this very instant, you would still be exactly the same elements and organic compounds you were one Nano-second before you died. You'd still contain all the vitamins, minerals, amino acids, water and solutions you did one second before you died. Everything before you died, would be exactly the same as it was the second after you died, except for the absence of one element. Do you know what that element is? It's the one and only thing that makes you dead. It's the one and only thing that, when put back, makes you alive again. The absence of this one element is the only thing that determines you being "alive" or "dead." The very instant you dropped dead, the one and only element missing from your body that was there just one millisecond before is, "electricity." When the electricity is gone, you're dead.

What is the first thing they use to jump start you when your heart stops? Electricity. Slap on the paddles, turn up the voltage, "clear" and wham-o, back to life, providing your battery is in good enough shape to hold a charge.

But, there is an important rule to remember: Though your cells exist in their own little, individual townships, just as every vessel must have a captain, they are programmed to listen to "one" voice, YOU! Be careful how you run your ship. Mutiny is always just around the corner. And that's what this book is all about, cleaning your ship from inside out and top to bottom, getting rid of all the crusty barnacles, sludge, gunk and critters that want to try and take over your ship. Its all about maintaining your vessel, stocking it with the proper supplies and keeping it sailing for as long as she can possibly sail.

Did you know: Under the Admiralty Laws of the Sea, all vessels are referred to as "She?"

So, now you are the Captain and keeper of an electrical-generating cellular community, floating in a pool of ether and electricity. Once in a while, a cell may ignore the command of the main voice, jump ship, venture out on its own and, "Houston, we have a problem." Dis-ease is born. This book will help you keep everybody, in line, working hard, on board and happy to be there. Happy sailing, Cap'n.'

EATING ELECTRICITY

Every well-structured organization must have at least some set of rules or guidelines to follow. Nature is one of the most complex organizational structures known. So, as we go along, I'm going to be suggesting rules that are important to remember and follow to help us keep our "Body, Mind and Spirit Organization" performing at the top of the charts and far longer than anyone ever anticipated possible.

First, let's talk a little more about electricity and **Rule #1**:

"You DO NOT live off the food you eat. You live off the electricity produced by the digestion of the food you eat."

Let's look at this one more time because its very important for you to understand. You want to eat "high-electricity" foods or foods with "high-energy" potential. I'll explain:

You are allotted just so much energy at any given time to perform all of your metabolic and physiological tasks like thinking, walking, talking, breathing, digesting, healing, etc. You might ask, "Why can't I just have some more energy? I already don't have enough to function as it is." The answer to that is: You <u>can</u> have more energy and I will show you how to get it. But first, I will show you, so you will understand, where the energy is going when you lose it.

The digestive process takes precedence over ALL other

metabolic functions because, obviously, this is where we get our nourishment. This is also where we are going to generate a lot of electricity. This is also one area to investigate where we may be losing energy as well.

What happens when we begin the digestive process? First of all, it takes massive amounts of energy to digest food. And remember, you are only allotted a certain amount of energy for the entire body. This is why all the other systems must temporarily give up their share of the energy so that we may digest the food. What this means is the immune system must give up its energy- or basically- shut down because of the importance of the fuel created during the digestive process. So, this means healing and repair jobs must be put on the back burner. After all, they, too, depend on the energy produced from the digestion of the newly consumed food.

What exactly happens with all this energy during digestion? Well, first of all, your body is set up with a digestive "supply-on-demand" system. This means, your pancreas and liver produce only the enzymes needed at that particular digestion event, no more, no less.

You don't have an enzyme pool with a bunch of extra enzymes just floating around waiting for some food to digest. The body doesn't know whether your next meal will be starchy, (amylase enzyme) fats, (lipase) proteins, (protease) or cellulose, (cellulase). We don't have enough room in our community for a pool to accommodate that many spare enzymes. This is the reason and necessity for the "demand enzyme" system. Make only what is needed, no more, no less.

So far, so good? We were about to make some energy here. Actually, we are about to <u>lose</u> some energy, first.

Let's say, you just sat down in front of a nice, juicy cut of prime-rib to watch, Downton Abbey. You take that knife and ever-so-expertly, carve that first tender, savory slice. Then, the juices begin to spill out onto your plate and into the potatoes. But you don't even care because the swirling, steaming, delightfully delectable, delicate aroma wraps around your olfactory senses, stimulating your endorphins and love is in the air. Its just so overwhelming, you can't get it into your mouth quickly enough.

(You don't even care that Mary Crawley's lover just dropped dead in her bed.)

You begin to chew and salivate. Its…heavenly, absolutely, heavenly. Aaaaah….!

Recalling our first rule about eating live, electrical foods, that delectable morsel of meat goes sliding down the fuel pipe. Remember now, this is a dead piece of meat that has no electrical potential what-so-ever because, why? Its dead! And not only that, its been cooked to well over 118 degrees Fahrenheit to kill all the parasites and bacteria, making it fit for human consumption. So, all the digestive enzymes that would otherwise have assisted with the digestion of this food have been cooked out and destroyed.

Now, when this dead piece of meat collides with your own digestive enzymes, which are already weakened from too many cooked foods, we don't generate a spark or even the slightest little puff of smoke. There has been no electricity produced and none of the original digestive food enzymes were left intact. So, after dinner, instead of being full of vigor and vitality, we feel listless and sleepy because all our reserve energy is being gobbled up by our digestive system. Then, to add to the already taxing process, we are having to produce 100% of the digestive enzymes needed to digest the stuff. And, to add insult to injury, our own digestive enzymes, being so weak from poor eating habits and out of range pH's, must be produced in excess. The existing ones just don't have the energy potential to do the job.

Next, let's metaphorically dump a whole bunch of salt on our already gaping wound as we probably didn't bother to chew our food up past the size of a golf-ball and barely small enough to swallow.

We take a big sigh, push ourselves away from the table, pat our belly and what do we want to do? We want to go lie down and take a nap. Why do we want to go lie down and take a nap?

Because no potential energy has been produced. In fact, we are about to lose even more energy. Why? Because no energy was produced during the meal and now we are going to take away even more from our already depleted well. We still must digest the food and that takes energy- lots of energy.

On the other hand, let's say you've been taking very good care of yourself, getting everything cleaned out and rebuilt with the proper nutrients and both your liver and pancreas are in top shape and producing little "monster enzymes"; ones that can digest the toughest of foes. They're ready to tear up everything in sight. Hold on now, 'cause we're about to **make** some energy!
(Move over, Nikola Tesla!)
Okay, let's say you went to the store, bought some nice, fresh, non-GMO, organic produce and made yourself a great-big healthy salad. You take a big bite of bright-green, raw and alive, organic broccoli, that still contains ALL its original enzymes. That broccoli will digest seventy to eighty percent on its own, without any other assistance. As it makes its way through your digestive system and collides with your little "monster enzymes," an explosion occurs, smoke billows and sparks fly. You have just created energy. You take another bite and another and another. With every bite you continue this relentless barrage of electrical explosions over and over again. Your body is getting stronger and stronger because you are building up reserve energy. And it's having time to repair and heal itself because of not having to make so many digestive enzymes. With continued eating of this electricity-producing food, you will build up such a reserve of energy, you couldn't possibly ever use it up!

You no longer need to sleep after dinner. You're ready to go shopping or hiking or biking or jogging or dancing. Baby, you're ready to rock 'n' roll all night!

Eat for electricity. Eat high electricity foods: raw vegetables and fruits, fresh juices, nuts, seeds and sprouts. Eat foods that haven't been cooked to death. Leave the original enzymes intact. With every bite, feel the power. Feel the electricity. You'll soon be feeling the lightning bolts shooting through your veins.

Feel alive! I'm not saying you have to be a vegetarian. I'm just saying eat more raw and lightly cooked foods to give your body a break. Let your immune system have more quality time for extended periods to heal and repair its Captain.

UNDERSTANDING THIS ENERGY

Let me start off by saying, "Every cell in your body and every organ comprised of those cells, has a specific ideal electrical frequency. In other words, every cell, organ and metabolic system in your body, has a perfect or specific electrical frequency produced when working properly.

Electrical frequencies are referred to in terms of Hertz (Hz) meaning cycles per second. The normal human body's working electrical frequency range is between 62 Hz to 68 Hz. If you were to hold a cup of coffee and measure electrical output, it would register around 58 Hz. If you would go one step further and take a sip of that coffee, it will immediately register about 52 Hz. That has drastically altered our electrical output. Colds invade and disease begins at 58 Hz, flu-like symptoms at 57 Hz, Candida at 55 Hz, Epstein Barr at 52 Hz and at 42 Hz we are overcome with cancer.

When a frequency starts drifting out of range, the organ, cell or system begins to fail. For example: the frequency of a healthy pancreas is 7.9 Hz (cycles per second). Around the age of twenty years or so, due to poor dietary habits and toxic accumulation, the pancreas begins to lose its electricity and drops to around 4.5 Hz. When this happens, swelling and disease are just around the corner.

How does this happen? From improper electrical stimuli or mineral imbalance. That's right, you haven't been feeding your body the right frequencies. Every element that goes in your body has an electrical frequency attached to it. Every time you eat, every supplement you take and every drink of water or whatever you drink, you are altering or re-adjusting your electrical frequencies.

This is a good time to introduce **Rule #2:**

"All diseases are caused by mineral imbalances, toxins or both."

This rule is very important. Here you will begin to see how toxins can block energy, and improper nutritional intake can under or over adjust a potential frequency. Here's an example:

Let's say your liver is giving you problems. Its not filtering toxins out of your blood properly, to the point you might even be turning yellow. Your nutrients aren't being picked up and sent where they should be going, and your blood oxygen isn't being made available at the cellular level. These are just a few of the over one thousand tasks your liver has to perform.

So, how do we go about fixing Mr. Liver? We first give him a good detox-cleansing. Then, we begin feeding the proper support calciums and nutrients. In essence, what are we doing? We are adjusting or tweaking the liver's electrical frequencies. Calciums adjust your liver frequencies. There are alkaline calciums to drive acidic frequencies or pH's into the proper range and acidic calcium to push the too alkaline frequencies toward a more acidic range. We will get more in depth on this subject a little later on. Right now, we are going to examine your "glowing-ness."

YOU'RE A LIGHT BULB

Your "aura" or more scientifically put, the luminescence of your "Electro-magnetic field," is the sum of all your body's electrical frequencies radiating outward. Just as the energy or luminescence from a light bulb cannot be contained within the bulb itself and radiates past the outer perimeter of the bulb, the electricity generated by the molecular movement inside your own body, intensifies and must radiate outward past your body's outer perimeter. You glow. A sick person will emit a very dull and weak aura, projecting only a few inches outward whereas, a healthy person's aura may radiate many feet away from the body.

Now, let's say your aura is radiating a nice, peaceful blue

color, except for one small gray area over your left temple. (Yes, auras can be seen by anyone who allows his or herself to do so, or by the use of Kirlian photography techniques.) What's causing this gray area to appear in this harmonious flow of the sum of all your body's frequencies? Proper frequencies are lacking in a certain group of cells or a specific system, from lack of proper minerals or toxic deposits interfering with or limiting their abilities to produce the proper frequencies.

How do we compensate or correct this problem? We first trace the gray area down through the energy meridians or acupuncture points this area crosses, determine what organs, system, or cells are associated with this meridian and ingest the missing electrical frequencies. An alternative practitioner may use electronic frequency generators, color therapy, sound therapy or a number of other modalities. Yes, every frequency resonates a color and an electrical frequency. Its ALL about electricity. A typical "A" note played on a piano would vibrate at 440 Hz. If you were able to observe this note through a spectrograph, it would also be producing a particular shade of emerald green color. Color, sound and electricity are ALL inner-changeable because they are all made up of electrical vibrations.

CHAPTER 2
THE CAUSE OF DISEASE

The cause of disease is not a "mystery" as modern medicine would have you believe. Temporary symptomatic suppressing prescriptions, or radical, surgical removal of diseased organs, comes nowhere near the cause or cure to any degree.

We seem to want to wait until disease has progressed to a recognizable form, until it has developed a definite pathology. In the meantime, we have sacrificed needless time and opportunity. We wait until we have symptoms, and this is surely the treatment we shall receive. To wait until symptoms appear is like locking the stable door after your horses have been stolen.

Modern medicine is based on science. Science is based on provable truth. If it is not provable truth, it is not science. Therefore, it is not true. Unfortunately, our medical scientific beliefs are that closed minded. The proof is in the pudding. If it works, it works. You don't need to have a degree to figure that one out.

"A closed mind should also keep a closed mouth."

Why would organized medicine want to pry into and expose the real cause of disease? To come to the realization of the causation and eradication of disease would largely eliminate the physician from our lives. This surely would not be the wish of the medical establishment. The community of "modern medicine."

What an oxymoron of a reference to the medical establishment we have constructed. We are a modern world with less than primitive techniques for curing the dis-eases of the human body. Did I say curing? My mistake. We aren't talking about ham. When was the last time you heard of anybody being "cured" of high blood pressure after being on their blood pressure meds for the last ten or fifteen years.? What about arthritis? What about gout? High cholesterol? COPD? Asthma? Depression? Diabetes? These are common, everyday ailments. You know the funny thing is, they have us actually believing they are doing the best things for us. The sad part of this egregious scenario is that they themselves think this is the actual truth. The doctors have been led to believe the same ambiguous lie that they are providing the most appropriate and effective treatment available. After all, they are trained in the world of "modern medicine."

The Common Wealth Fund Report ranks the United States, boasting as the most sophisticated medical system in the world, at number 37, IN THE WORLD. Maybe that could be the explanation of why medicine kills over 370,000 patients a year. That's right. Our modern medical world is the third leading cause of death, just behind heart disease and cancer.

If you were to visit your doctor and say, "Hey, Doc, I think I've got high cholesterol. What do you think I should do?" Do you think your doctor is going to say, "Do a lemon-water fast, take five tablespoons of lecithin and five garlic cloves for fourteen days, cut down on your consumption of animal flesh, come back and see me in two weeks and it will be normal"? After he's done testing, he's going to write you a prescription for a lifetime setup of pills that will create yet another set of problem side effects that will necessitate yet another regime of more "advanced" pharmaceuticals and on and on and on.

On behalf of my patients that are doctors and nurses and the majority of the doctors practicing medicine, I wish they would quite referring to it as "practicing."

I will answer the question I have been asked many times: "Why do they keep doing this same inadequate protocol over and over?" Because this is what they have been taught. This is what they have also been led to believe. There is also one more angle to this abstract picture, and I know this because I have verified it with my patients. The medical doctors are on a quota set by the pharmaceutical industry. If the doctor does not meet that quota each month, he or she is visited by a pharmaceutical rep and informed that if those prescriptions are not brought up to the designated specifications, if that quota is not met, they will lose their medical license. That puts a lot at stake.

Here's the other thing. I have been approached in the past by medical universities asking me to assist with patients suffering incurable diseases when the physicians were unable to exhibit any signs of improvement. Unfortunately, they were not allowed to participate in my methodologies for fear of being disbarred from the medical field. Our medical system is full of doctors that want to do more. They want more knowledge to truly help their patients. They see that there is more knowledge. Its just not within their allowed protocols. Their hands are tied by Big Pharma.

Did you know, in China, the doctor would be paid until the person became ill. Makes a lot more sense and quite an incentive to get the patient back on their feet as soon as possible. Just as Las Vegas wasn't built on winners, the pharmaceutical industry doesn't get fat on healthy humans.

Except for the time I was suppose to be born dead, I have never been to a medical doctor in my life, and I actually didn't make that appointment.

This passage, speaking in reference to the mainstream medical field is amusing to say the least. In Doctor William Hay's book written in 1929, he quotes,

"...the light gives evidence it is about to break, and if official medicine will not harken to the voice of protest on the question of adequate training, the attitude of the enlightened public will force change within a very few more years, else the medical colleagues will have to close their door."

My, haven't we come a long way? If only Doctor Williams could see things now. Every show on T.V is interrupted by the next perfect pill for all your needs. "It may cause headaches, diarrhea, nausea, vomiting, sexual disfunction, birth defects, damage to your liver, kidneys, cause lymphoma and even death. Ask your doctor if its right for you." What better sleep aid could you ask for. With all those wonderful thoughts beating around in your head, *have a nice nap!* What do we they think we are, stupid? The pitiful answer to that rhetorical question is, "YES" to the tune of 400 billion dollars a year, stupid! After all they tell us, all these bad side effects, (even death) they still prescribe them and the worst part is, people still take them. The only person these pills are right for are "Doctor Cadillac" and the pharmaceutical moguls. Its about wealth not health. Its quite sad, the moral has been replaced by the dollar.

Instead of taking pills that are going to cause side effects and possibly going to kill you, and most often are not going to remedy the malady you started taking them for in the first place, why don't you just stop doing what gave you the problem to begin with? If you hit your thumb with a hammer, are you gonna hit it again to make it quite hurting? Does that sound any dumber than having a simple illness and taking something to cure it that may kill you? Well, that would surely eradicate the problem now, wouldn't it?

Dr. George W. Crile states, *"A death from so called natural causes is merely the end-point of progressive acid saturation."* In other words, from the continual over-consumption of acid-forming foods; concentrated meat proteins, greasy fried foods, sodas, processed sugars, coffee, alcohol, food additives and food colorings, our body can adjust and compensate no more and it finally shuts down. What causes this acid saturation? Too much acid-forming foods without proper drainage of the colon. Death by natural causes is caused by improper drainage and acid.

A QUICK pH REFRESHER

Remember this:

1. On the pH scale 7.0 pH is neutral, neither acid nor alkaline.
2. Tap water is kept at or around 7.0 pH or neutral.
3. If you were to drink 8 oz. of soda, being quite acidic at 2.5 pH, it would take thirty-two 8 oz glasses of 10 pH water to neutralize the acid in the soda. So, you would have to be adding some high doses of pH drops in your water to achieve an alkalinity level of 10 pH. Wouldn't want to do that for very long.

Coffee and alcohol both hover right around that same pH range and wine is about 3.0 pH. And since I brought it up, its been recently discovered that 2 ounces of wine can double a woman's risk of developing breast cancer. Better off getting your anti-oxidants from grape juice. Pour it in a wine glass and pretend it's romantic. No, I'm not picking on you ladies. Wine and alcohol with men can cause erectile disfunction and impotence and though a small amount may give you confidence, it can also quickly disillusion and even put an end to your romantic evening. Grape juice with a little baking soda: tastes like grape soda pop and will boost your voltage!

SO WHEN DOES DISEASE START?

"Disease begins only when the body loses its ability to make healthy cells that work."

And death occurs only when this condition cannot be reversed.

I will continue to repeat this mantra until you have it thoroughly burned into your brain. How does disease originate in a body created and brought into this world in supposedly normal conditions? At what age does disease begin?

When one is born of fairly healthy parents, chances are that baby is created perfect. This is Nature's original blueprint of things to be. Nature is perfect. It doesn't make mistakes. If someone is born with inadequacies, somewhere along the way, humans got involved. It may have been done in a totally innocent and unaware means. The parents had poor diets, or their parents had poor diets. It may have been an environmental toxin ingestion somewhere along the way. It might trace back to an event several generations back that caused, not a genetic weakness, (which in actuality, accounts for only 4% of true genetic illnesses) but an **"inherent weakness"** such as a re-occurring organ weakness that transferred down to the new generation brought on by nutritional deficiencies, not haywire genes. I will explain this shortly. It might have been the result of medical error such as side effects from medication prescribed during the gestation period or years before the mother ever became pregnant. It literally may be residue left in the liver from medications given to the mother as a child. Nature doesn't make mistakes, humans do.

For now, let's say we are born with all our usual parts and our organs are working fine. We may have an adjustment to make here and there but our body chemistry has all the organic chemical compounds in perfect proportions that a good, healthy human is supposed to have. All-in-all, the Creator has made us a pretty good package, packed our bags well and provided us with all the essentials we will need to embark on this new "Journey of Life."

Where does disease begin? On the spiritual and emotional realms it begins at conception. (more on that, later) Right now, we're discussing the physical level. Obviously, the health of both the parents plays a definite role in the original ingredients that went into the recipe. But during the gestation period, it pretty much all depends on the mother's health and her ability to remain in a healthy state until the birthing. The diet and the substances being passed through the placenta to the fetus, be they nutrients or toxins, are writing the outcome of the story.

Babies born with so called "inherent weaknesses" (again, not to be confused with genetic weakness) may be traced back to either parent, or even further. I would like to shed a different beam of light from a different angle on this concept.

Let's take a baby born with weak kidneys. If, during the gestation period, the mother herself is suffering from kidney deficiencies, as simple as dehydration, the mother's body will actually pull energy from the fetus' own kidneys, as a natural compensation for survival, pre-programmed by nature, leaving the new born with weakened kidneys.

This is an example of an "inherent weakness," a weakness possibly on the mineral level as opposed to a weakness caused by an actual weak, malfunctioning or missing gene. This is not the fault, or a deliberate decision made by the mother. She would unselfishly give up her own kidneys or give her life for her baby. It's Nature, doing what it is programmed to naturally do. It's the natural "law of selection." It has nothing to do with ethics or morals or the lack thereof. It's simply an innate quality control system adapted for enabling Nature to continue producing her perfect line of products.

What the mother could have done was to make a conscious effort to change her diet, to repair and support her own body, strengthen her immune system and be in the most optimal shape possible for supporting two bodies. Without proper nutrients, in ample quantities, the mother will run short and not be able to provide for the developing fetus. Nothing comes from nothing and Nature cannot make the mother give up what she does not have. A toxic mother can only produce toxic milk.

I know, it would appear I am laying all this on the mother. Dads and Dads-to-Be, you have responsibilities as well. You can research the best possible diets and supplements for the mother and assist and support with a healthy regime that will benefit both she and the baby to be. If you smoke, don't do it around the mother-to-be. Share the healthy eating habits with her. Support, support, support! That's the kind of love she needs now.

After the child is born, let's assume he or she is perfect, as we know they ALL are, no matter what. But let's just say this particular baby is an exceptionally healthy baby. First thing we will do is try and feed it (hopefully breastfeed). Then after a short while, for some unknown reason, it begins to cry. Our first assumption is it must be hungry again. So, we feed it some more and it starts to regurgitate the milk.

Now remember, a newborn has only enough digestive enzymes in its mouth to break down mother's milk. None exist yet in the digestive tract. Then, we feed it some more! After all, babies are suppose to be fat and squishy. Then starts the diarrhea, the baby's crying, and we're panicking. How do we respond? By what we've been programmed to believe. Must be hungry. Needs more food! Not so.

These are sure signs of over-nourishment. Too much feeding. Thus begins the "poor drainage" syndrome. The body tries to adjust and compensate. As the intestines start to spasm from exhaustion, a colic condition begins. Now, its time to go to the doctor. He administers some medicine for the baby's condition. You have now compromised the baby's immune system for the first time with a synthetic, non-organic material and so begins the decline of that baby's immune system.

Next, the baby is graduated to cow's milk. **Did you know**: bovine milk is 3 times the protein concentration than human mother's milk? It was designed to support and develop an animal the size of a car.

Now, the human mind wants to think; protein, one of the great building blocks. More has to be better. Not always the case. Excess animal protein is very hard on the kidneys of even grownups. A newborn doesn't have a chance at processing cow milk. Goat's milk is a far better choice (if it doesn't taste like a wet dog smells.)

If a child does not die by the age of ten, a tolerance for toxins develops. Acute eruptions of diarrhea, toxic headaches, vomiting, are evidence to lack of the ability to dump toxic waste matter, as the body slowly becomes "auto-intoxicated." (poisoned) This is the first sign of body's decline, the **beginning of disease.**

The baby then has solid foods added to its diet in the way of concentrated meat proteins, harsh starches and more cow's milk. Protein is used for reconstruction of broken-down muscle tissue. Setting the meat aside, a baby could never use up the amount of protein the average child consumes in cow's milk alone. One egg a day is far too much protein, as well as is one quart of dairy milk for any child less than eight or ten years of age,

This excess protein puts major stress on the baby's digestive system as well as the liver and kidneys. A child's liver is not fully developed until age twelve and should not even be eating meat of any sort until it reaches at least the age of two years. Again, the not completely developed child has just enough ptyalin or starch-digesting saliva enzyme to break down milk-sugar and nothing more. Harsher sugars are therefore dumped into the stomach, unprocessed and have no provisions for further breakdown. The result is "acid fermentation." We now have our liver and digestive tract under great stress, and the acid fermentation results in gas buildup leading to stomach and bowel pains. That can even make grown-ups cry.

DEATH BY NATURAL CAUSES

Habits developed before the seventh year are most likely to be for life. We develop, or continue, our learned "inherited diet," continuing to pollute our bodies with toxic meats, fried foods, processed sugars, preservatives, food coloring, bleached-white flour, too much dairy, too much gluten and we find we are not having bowel-movements but once a day or less.

I want to point out; one daily bowel movement does not constitute diarrhea! So, if the food isn't coming out, where is it going? Well, the answer to that question isn't a pleasant one. It is laying in the intestines, laying in the colon, putrefying and oozing toxic gases and sewage into the bloodstream, auto-intoxicating one's entire system and creating a totally "acidic" and polluted environment.

Did you know: our blood visits every part of our body <u>every three hours</u> including the intestines. Whatever is laying in there, gets picked up by the blood on its visit. And along its journey around the body, begins depositing its treasures from the intestines into every organ and system of our body. Before long, your sewer system has grown outside its containment area, the intestines, and is now everywhere. We start to feel tired and sluggish. The body does its best to deal with this growing situation, and the crud continues to accumulate. But there is only so much it can do and a certain length of time it can hold on and soon, begins to break down. Trash Union went on strike!

We begin to have irritable bowels, developing signs of diverticulitis, arthritis and high blood pressure. Our "bad" cholesterol level begins to sky-rocket. Then, here comes our first heart attack. I say first heart attack because if something is not changed, you can expect another after another until it refuses to tick any longer.

After a few years of blood pressure and cholesterol medicines, the liver begins to shut down. Soon, everything begins to follow suit, because as one organ begins to fail, the organs on either side must take up the slack until they, themselves, begin to fail and one by one start shutting down.

Our body was trying to tell us something with that acute bout with diarrhea several years back, followed by the acid-reflux that began preventing us from a good night's sleep. But we just didn't listen. We need to learn to listen to our bodies. Listen, before they re-section your colon or strip out your leg arteries and transplant them into your heart.

Besides learning to love, maybe one of the main purposes of the human's existence here on earth, is to learn the use of the foods prepared by the Creator, in their natural form, and overcome so called "Death by Natural Causes."

YOUR INHERITED DISEASE OR INHERITED DIET?

Have you inherited all your family's diseases? No. You have inherited what I call the "Inherited Diet." In other words, you have inherited the poor eating habits that your parent's inherited, passed on from their parent's parents and so on right on down the line. Is all of this starting to make sense yet? Heart disease runs in your family? Trace it back and you will find generation after generation of over-consumption of animal fats, high salt and grease. Does high cholesterol run in your family? More than likely, so do foods high in saturated fats, along with poor digestive practices. Do you want to pass that on to your children and the next generation, or do you want to stop it right here and now?

CHAPTER 3
JUST WHAT IN THE pH ARE YOU TALKING ABOUT?

Suppose I told you, you can actually immune yourself from ever getting sick again in your life. I'm about to simplify and clarify a very complex and confusing subject that can do just that. And that is, the delicate balance between the acid and alkaline levels of your body, their effects on your organs and the symptomatic patterns associated with each one.

Let me start off by saying this subject plays one of the most important roles in keeping your body healthy, functioning to its full capacity and disease-free. Understand this, and you will hold the key to the Universe's greatest secret to human physical health and longevity.

Before we go any further, I would like to say, this chapter is going to expound upon the rather incomplete information or semi-misconceptions of pH balancing that have been continuously pass from book to book, and over the internet, leaving very large voids of knowledge on acid/alkaline balancing. The result could lead to a person not reaching the potential state of health he or she has been hoping to achieve. You can't just stick a pH strip in your mouth, make it turn blue and think all your problems are going to go away. There's much more to it than that.

The theory goes, periodically put a pH test strip or (litmus paper) on your tongue. Then, through various means from supplements to high alkalinity water, try to make your body as alkaline as you can get it because disease can't thrive in an alkaline environment. In theory this information is almost entirely true. As you continue through this chapter, you will begin to see why I say "almost." It is, however, somewhat inaccurate and incomplete. It is also not the way to achieve optimal homeostasis (balance) of the body. After reading this chapter, you will understand how to achieve the perfect balance of ALL your physiological functions and obtain the most optimal state of health you can possibly achieve.

If you would like to skip this chapter for the lack of need for technical information, I suggest you go on to the summary at the end of this chapter. However, I highly suggest you stay with us and at least attempt to learn this magical key to your health. If not, just wait for us there at the summary. We'll be along shortly.

For the rest of us that continue down the perilous and unrelenting "I need to know" pathway," let us begin. I hope to keep everyone entertained and on board. It may get a little technical at times, but I will try to make it as understandable and boring-free as possible. If you do have any questions, please, just hold up your hand.

First of all, what is the pH and why is it so important? The term pH stands for "potential hydrogen" which is, "a measurement of the particular amount of hydrogen atoms in the substance being measured." It is also a title interchangeable with the term "voltage." When the pH changes, the voltage changes. More on that subject in my last book "The Human Repair Manuel."

In actuality, the pH scale, by which we gauge pH, is a measurement of resistance or friction. When the pH moves toward the acidic range, what is actually taking place is an increase in potential energy flow because there is a decreasing resistance to the electrical flow. As this electrical flow increases there is an automatic increase in magnetism. Now, if the pH begins to move in the opposite direction towards the alkaline range, there is a decrease in energy or electrical flow potential because of the increased resistance. As expected, there is a decrease in magnetism due to the decreased electrical flow.

That all sounded a little on the complicated side and borderline "boring." Let me set up a visual here and it will make this all so much clearer. Very lightly, place your palms together. Now, without applying any pressure, begin rubbing your palms. Okay, speed up faster and faster until you can rub no faster. What you will notice is you can rub really fast but are generating very little heat, due to the fact there is no friction being created. No resistance, no friction. No friction, no heat. This would represent an <u>acidic</u> constitution. The person is fast and cold, possibly a workaholic but is the first person to complain of being cold. There is lack of heat friction, due to having too little alkaline calcium or too much acidic calcium, however you want to see it.

Now, we are going to rub our hands again. This time start out fast and slowly begin to apply pressure between your palms creating resistance. You will immediately notice slowing down and heat beginning to develop. This represents an alkaline constitution. This person is always hot because of the friction heat being generated but is also slower than the acidic person because of decreased magnetism due to decreased energy flow. So there is less energy potential, due to too much alkaline calcium and not enough acidic calcium.

So, in summary, an acidic person is fast and cold while an alkaline person is slow and hot.

One more way to look at it is this: (you can actually visualize this instead of actually doing it and save yourself a mess of cleaning water up) Take a piece of pipe, tilt it to at least a 45-degree angle. Now. Pour some water down the pipe. The water runs as fast out the exit end as it was going through the opening.

Now, glue a few marbles inside the pipe at various positions as not to stop the flow completely.(We'll call these alkaline calcium) What you should observe now is the water coming out of the pipe is slower than the water going in. We have added resistance. We have slowed the flow, while decreasing the potential energy flow of the water.

This is what happens when we adjust frequencies or pH's. We would add alkaline forming calciums to the system to slow it down and bring it within an acceptable or targeted alkaline range. Likewise we would add acidic calciums if the body were too alkaline. In dealing with calciums in the body, acidic calciums create less resistance and cause energy to flow through the body faster and increase the body's magnetism. Alkaline calciums create resistance, therefor slowing down electrical flow while decreasing magnetism. So, pH is not only a measurement of electrical flow, but also a measurement of magnetism. Also, alkaline energy flows <u>upwards</u> towards the upper parts of the body, while acidic energy flows <u>downwards</u> towards the feet.

Okay, using this new information, it's time to put it together and make our first diagnosis. What causes restless-leg syndrome? You nailed it, too acid. All the energy is flowing downward and reaching the intersection all at the same time with nowhere to go. This person also may experience hot feet until they remove their shoes, as the shoes are acting like capacitors and storing heat energy from too much acidic energy flow all at once. Starting to see how it all works?

For point of reference on the pH scale: **pure sulfuric acid** represents the extreme acid end of the scale at 00 pH. In pure sulfuric acid, electricity can travel at the speed of light. This makes sulfuric acid an ideal conductor of electricity. On the extreme opposite, or alkaline end of the scale is **Pure Calcium**, with a pH of 14 and is considered a "non-conductor" of electrical current because of its vary high resistance.

We are going to be dealing with four basic areas of pH; blood, urine, saliva and body tissue. Blood and most of the tissues of the body hover right around 7.4 pH which is slightly alkaline.
The urine and saliva pH's can very greatly during the day and can change radically by what we eat or drink.

Did you know: Simply getting angry, sad or upset can immediately drop you pH's by two or three points?

Did you know: According to statistics, America is one of the angriest countries on the planet? We are also one of the most acidic countries. Any correlation?

According to Carey Reams, a biologist who developed the RBTI, Urine/Saliva test, claims the optimal urine/saliva pH's for the human body to be 6.4 pH, which is slightly on the alkaline side. As you recall, cells need a working pH of 7.35 to 7.45 pH which also translates into -20 mV and -25 mV (millivolts or 1000th of a volt).

Here is where it gets a little confusing and I will be attempting to eliminate this confusion. I have been performing Reams urine/ saliva testing for over twenty years and have seen it work miraculously, especially concerning medical non-diagnosable maladies. While the cells need a pH of 7.4 pH, strangely enough, the metabolic functions of the body, seem to perform much more efficiently at 6.4 pH again, which is slightly acidic. With the digestive enzymes being more efficient, the overall working energy of the body is optimal, and the healing time is increased greatly. This is contrary to what you see on the internet and what your doctor has been taught in medical school.

So, here's the deal, 7.4 pH or -22.5 mV is ideal for your cells to perform. These are the cells that make up the tissues of the body. However, our metabolic functions are optimal at 6.4 pH. In fact: All biological life has the most optimal working energy at 6.4 to 6.5 pH. If you were to measure the pH of the healthiest plant in your garden, you would find it to be 6.5 pH. If you were to measure the unhealthiest, bug-infested plant you find its pH to be 6.0 pH or less. Your urine number measures what minerals you lack or have an overabundance of, while your saliva number is a measurement of the strength in your liver produced digestive enzymes. Your saliva is a direct connection to your liver.

I'm going to let all that be for now. If you want to pursue and learn more about Reams urine and saliva testing, you can research it on your own, It would take far too long and complicate the idea of simplifying this whole subject.

With that all said and out of the way, I am going to attempt to simply this whole ordeal. On the pH scale, from 0 acidic to 14 alkaline and 7.0 pH being the middle or neutral zone, we can get down to making easy sense of all this pH talk. Anything above the neutral 7.0 pH range is alkaline whereas, anything below 7.0 pH is acidic. It doesn't matter how far above or below, it's still either alkaline or acidic.

So, here comes **rule #3**:

"Acid breeds disease."

Any time your body becomes too acidic, you become a breeding ground for all types of disease. Every opportunistic germ, bacteria, mold, yeast fungus and virus in your body is just waiting for this opportune moment when your pH levels drop, and your immune system is weakened. Because that's what happens when we become too acidic. Our immune system begins breaking down no longer able to keep up with its tasks and begins to surrender to this out-of-control germ-breeding frenzy. Now, we're sick. It could be just a common cold, or it could be something more serious such as an auto-immune disease. In any event, we are acidic and ill.

On the other hand, or the other spectrum of the pH scale, germs cannot thrive in an alkaline environment. Alkalinity is very unfavorable to a germ. Their electrical frequencies are lowered, and they revert to a depressed state, basically laying dormant and unable to reproduce. They are kept in check.

But, let's not get carried away with this concept and think, "Wow, I'll just pour a bunch of alkaline water drops in my water, or get an alkaline water making machine, get my whole body really, really alkaline, kill all the little critters and never have to worry again. I will live forever!" Unfortunately, that's not the correct solution. You see, there are symptomatic patterns associated with both the acidic and alkaline constitution and the more extreme the pH direction, the more severe the symptoms. There are just as many dis-eases caused by being too alkaline as there are, too acidic. Here is a comparative list of ailments or dis-eases caused by either being too acidic or too alkaline. We will start with being too acidic first and remember, the more extreme into the pH range, the more drastic or severe the symptoms or reactions will be.

Here are the possibilities of the Acidic constitution; both urine and saliva below 7.0 pH:

1. Digestion becomes too fast even to the point of diarrhea.
2. Colitis and Crone's disease are favorable.
3. The bone loss is in the direction of osteoporosis. Deterioration can be especially pronounced in the bone structure supporting the teeth. Decay can remain minimal.
4. The left side of the body is the weakest with curvature of the spine pulling to the right side or strong side.
5. Your right leg will be shorter than your left.
6. You will tend to cross your right leg over your left.
7. There will usually be a lot of leg cramping, joint and bone aches as well as discomfort below the waist.
8. Dry skin and skin rashes.
9. Tendency to be very nervous.
10. Restless leg syndrome.
11. Fungus infections can become a problem.
12. Severe vitamin C, D and B-12 deficiencies.
13. Cells become more concentrated in shape, meaning areas of the body will change shape and texture, become harder and unable to function properly.
14. The perfect host for germs, viruses and bacteria.

These are just a few of the symptomatic patterns of the acidic constitution and as you will see, as I said before, extreme alkalinity can pose just as many symptomatic patterns and is NOT the answer. Here are the pattern symptomatics of an overly alkaline constitution. And as you might have guessed, some symptoms will be just the opposite of those of the acidic constitution. Here they are:

1. Pattern for constipation
2. System becomes overloaded with toxins from stored metabolic waste of cell function and bowel re-absorption

of putrefactive waste.

3. Parasites likely present as free room and board are being provided.
4. Aggravated spinal disk deterioration.
5. Deterioration of cartilage.
6. Upper respiratory, sinus and lymph congestion.
7. May be prone to lung infections.
8. Body odors from breath to bowel gas.
9. With age, the abdomen may become distended.
10. Over production of Vitamin D causing skin pigmentation problems
11. Skin tumors and lesions may be problematic.
12. May have excessive tooth decay.
13. Right side of the body is the weaker with strong tendency of developing curvature of the spine to the left, as the body pulls towards the stronger right side.
14. Blood pressure can be affected.
15. Tends to cross left leg over right and right leg being the shorter.
16. Possible developments of stones (i.e., kidney)

As you can see, there are many problems associated with an over-alkaline constitution as well. But, lucky for us, scientists like Dr. Carey Reams and others have figured most of it out and have provided us with a direction in which road to travel. Now, its up to each one of us to stay on that road. Like I said, I have been performing Reams testing for 20+ years and it never ceases to amaze me how the pH's of just the urine and saliva can divulge so much information about a patient. I have had patients think I'm psychic because of the information I can tell them about themselves from this simple test. But, its all in the numbers and learning the interpretation. I have had patients try to convince me they were doing exactly as I instructed them to do and their numbers were just not responding. Every time after retesting, they would admit, okay, maybe I didn't do everything I was suppose to do. The numbers don't lie.

THE EFFECTS OF pH AND CALCIUMS ON THE LIVER

Okay, one more topic before we put it all together and make incredibly enlightened sense of all this information on: How pH's and calciums affect the liver's ability to perform its functions.

Your liver is one of the most important organs in your body. Sure, we need the heart to pump the blood, the lungs to breathe and move the air and provide us with oxygen, the brain to act as our major control center. But, the liver has more responsibilities and more tasks to perform than any other organ in your body. Three of the more than one thousand tasks required by the liver are nutritional distribution, blood filtration and digestion regulation. Right now, these are the three liver tasks we are most concerned with.

Did you know: if the liver can't find a certain needed element in the blood, it will actually eat a part of itself, find and extract the mineral or vitamin needed, send it to the area in need, then regenerate that part of itself it just consumed? Kind of like a lizard swallowing then re-growing its tail back. It is one of the only organs that is recognized as actually capable of regeneration. This is why the liver retains every element needed for the human body within its tissues for just this sort of emergency. The liver is the nutritional distribution center for the entire body and if the brain says, "We need more potassium to the heart," it's the liver's job to acquire and supply this nutrient, being the element storage center. Its kind of like the Amazon distribution center.

Another important factor to remember is that every minuscule particle of matter, mineral, chemical, medicine and toxin that enters your bloodstream enters your liver, and many of the residues are trapped and left behind to accumulate and pull the liver's vital energy force down. This is why many of the drugs advertisements warn, "May cause liver damage" or "Do not use if you have been diagnosed with a liver problem."

Let's talk about the electrical frequencies of the liver and the effects of calciums on these frequencies. Here is where you will see the importance of the liver's frequencies and the digestive process.

At this point I want to make it clear when I am referring to pH's in regards to urine/saliva or (liver) numbers, I am speaking in terms of "electro-magnetic energy potential" and not "acid or alkaline ash" as with foods. We're talking pure energy now.

If you will recall, the symptomatic patterns of both acid and alkaline constitution had a huge effect on the digestive process. This has to due with the liver and the energy potential your body is producing. Au contraire, to popular suggestion, we actually want to keep the urine and saliva pH's at 6.4, which is slightly acidic. This puts the liver on its perfect electrical frequency for optima function.

Interestingly, all biological life seems to have its best electrical flow and magnetism at this 6.4 pH resistance point, the "ideal range."

This may sound confusing and quite contradictory to everything I have said so far, and that you have been previously told by the internet. But, by the time we get finished here, and we are almost to that point, you will see and understand the logic and how it all works. I promise!

TUNE UP THAT RADIO

For the time being, let's look at the liver as if it were a radio receiver. Now, there are certain bands of radio waves that our liver/radio is able to pick up. However, our radio is losing its ability to pick up certain radio frequencies or in actuality, nutrients. Our liver/radio is slowly losing its ability to pick up let's say, station vitamin C from the blood. Why? Because the liver is starting to fade out of its ideal frequency range of 6.4 pH making it unable to recognize and pull vitamin C from the blood. Similar to going down in a valley and losing radio reception, when your liver gets too far away from its ideal frequency range, it will completely lose its ability to recognize any nutrients, or in the case of radios, it is unable to pick up any stations. It will perceive these substances, in the case of vitamin C, as foreign objects and send them to the kidney's for extraction. It will also do the same thing to cells that are passing through.

You see, when the liver gets too far out of its ideal frequency range, it loses its ability to recognize any nutrient or substance, good or bad. This affects the internal aging process or the breaking down of the body at the cellular level. Our liver has developed temporary "dementia." We can take all the vitamins in the world, by the mega-gramfuls, and not one milligram or microgram will be pulled from the blood by the liver and distributed to the body's needs. We just end up with expensive urine.

This reason being is why many persons don't see results from the vitamin supplements they ingest. "But I was told these were the best on the market." Doesn't matter.

We can't use a screwdriver to adjust our liver/radio so," How do we fix it," you ask? Calcium. The liver is reliant on calcium. What was pulling the liver's frequencies out of range in the first place was the incorrect balance between acidic and alkaline calciums. "What do you mean, acid and alkaline calciums?" Again, you ask. The majority of people have never heard that there are at least eight different types of calcium used by the body. Some are alkaline forming, and some are acidic in nature. Some move the pH range of the urine in either direction and some respond to the saliva pH range direction.

Remember I said, every element has an electrical frequency attached to it? So, by determining what calciums are lacking in the liver, we can ingest the proper type and dosage of calcium/s and thereby tweak and adjust the liver's frequencies, restoring its functions back to optimal potential. There, that wasn't so bad after all.

PUTTING THE PIECES OF THE pH PUZZLE IN PLACE

Now, for the fun stuff. I've heard tell, if your urine and saliva pH's ever reach the same level, YOU WILL DIE! If this is the case, I have a lot of dead patients running around enjoying life.

This just simply, isn't true. In actuality, identical urine and saliva pH is what you are ideally wanting to achieve. You see, the further apart the spread between the urine and saliva numbers, the more eruptive your digestive system becomes (i.e., gas, bloating, pain, etc.)

Let's go back to our original four pH categories, blood, urine, saliva and tissue. First we have our blood, which we won't even worry about, as it is controlled by metabolic processes and enzymes and hovers right around 7.4 pH. What we are primarily concerned with are the remaining three categories.

First, we have the urine and saliva. We'll double them up and call them the "liver" numbers. Next, the tissues, or your actual body, your exterior (skin, muscles, etc.) From now on, when I'm speaking of keeping you at an alkaline pH, (anything above 7.0) I am referring to your body tissues.

We actually want our liver numbers or urine/saliva to be on the slightly acidic side at respectively, 6.4 pH. Remember, 7.0 pH as being neutral. This is the ideal working pH range, creating the perfect electrical frequencies or magnetic configuration for optimal function of the liver. When combining the ideal range numbers of your carbohydrates, urine/saliva pH, electrolyte level, cell debris and ureas or (nitrogen), your body will be functioning at the most optimal level possible. Which is a whole other book in itself. Maybe in the future?

Here is a list of the different types of calcium used tin adjusting the liver pH and frequencies:

Those of the acidic type:
1. Phosphate calcium
2. Sulphate calcium
(calcium lactate)
Alkaline calcium types:
1. Carbonate calcium (Tums)
2. Carbonate Magnesium (Dolomite)
3. Calcium Oxides (Citrate, gluconate)

4. Calcium Hydroxides (these build bones)
5. Calcium Hydrate (Lyme Water)

Its true, you will be obtaining these types of calciums through food in gestation. However, not in large enough quantities needed to move specific urine and saliva pH numbers in a particular direction, be they too far out of range of 6.4 pH.

In final, let's talk about the last category, your body tissue. <u>You</u> are about to become <u>immuned</u>. Remember, the body regulates the blood pH's. The liver's (urine/saliva) pH's are adjusted with calcium. So how do we adjust and maintain our tissue or body pH's? Food. This is the key which unlocks the secret door. Food combinations that provide the proper balance of acid-forming and alkaline-forming ash. When you get your tissue pH's at 7.4 pH, germs will run from you. You could eat a bowl of the flu and will not be able to get sick. Germs hate alkalinity. We will talk in depth on this subject in the 80/20 Alkaline Eating chapter.

IN SUMMARY

Okay, those of you who jumped off at the last stop, good to have you back on board with us. You missed quite a ride. Here is the summary of keeping the pH's of the body in perfect balance:
1. Your liver pH is adjusted with calcium. (potential energy)
2. Your body tissue is regulated with foods (sugar ashes)
3. Keep your body tissue at 7.4 pH for immunity to illness.
4. Keep urine and saliva pH's at 6.4 for optimal liver, digestive and body energy potential. Use pH strips or pH meter for testing.
5. Keep your body tissue at 7.4 pH by eating the 80/20 alkaline diet. Meaning, eat 80 percent alkaline-forming foods and 20 percent acid-forming foods. Again, this will be covered in detail in the Alkaline Diet chapter.

CHAPTER 4

WHAT AM I MADE OF?

Your body is made of approximately: 75 trillion cells, 206 bones, 639 muscles, 8 major glands, 31 types of organs, 60,000 miles of blood vessels, 45 miles of nerves, over 300,000 types of enzymes, numerous proteins, 22 amino acids, 40 liters of fluid, 5.5 liters of blood, 35,000 genes, 3 million pain receptors, 500,000 touch receptors, 30,000 heat receptors and enough DNA strands to go from here to the sun and back 66.47 times (that's about 6 trillion-503 billion miles, if stretched end to end) and all comprised of the following sixteen basic elements and 120 trace minerals.

Here is a list of the sixteen biochemicals that make up the human body, going in order of greatest percentage to least percentage. Weight measurements are of a 160-pound man or woman.

Element	Percentage	Weight
1. Oxygen	72	90 lb
2. Carbon	13.50	36 lb
3. Hydrogen	9.10	14 lb
4. Nitrogen	2.50	3 lb 8 oz
5. Calcium	1.30	3 lb 12 oz
6. Phosphorous	1.15	1 lb 4 oz
7. Sulphur	0.147 6	3.5 oz
8. Sodium	0.10	2.5 oz
9. Chlorine	0.085	4 oz
10. Fluorine	0.080	2 oz
11. Potassium	''0.026	3 oz
12. Magnesium	0.012	1.5 oz
13. Iron	0.010	1/6 oz
14. Silicon	0.0002	1/4 oz
15. Iodine, copper, lead, aluminum	0 (trace)	Trace
16. Manganese	trace	'Trace

CHEMICAL ELEMENTS OF PARTS OF THE BODY

(This can be very useful when determining weaknesses or deficiencies in a particular organ, part or system.)

Body Proteins: Carbon, hydrogen, nitrogen, phosphorus, iron and Sulphur

Body Fat: Carbon, hydrogen and oxygen

Percent of water in tissues: Fat 20%, blood 80%, bone 25%, liver 70%, muscles 75%, brain 85%, nerves 70%

Muscles: Potassium, magnesium, chlorine, manganese, calcium, selenium, phosphorus

Teeth and Bones: Calcium, magnesium, phosphorus, fluorine, copper, silicon

Joints and Ligaments: Sodium, iron and manganese

Hair and Nails: Silicon, Sulphur, iron, zinc and chlorine

Skin: Silicon, sodium, Sulphur, copper and manganese

Brain and Nerves: Phosphorus, magnesium, sodium, potassium, Sulphur, iodine, calcium and manganese

Heart: Potassium, magnesium, calcium, phosphorus, iron

Blood: Iron, copper, sodium, zinc, potassium, and calcium

Blood Vessels: Magnesium, Sulphur and silicon

Liver: Zinc, selenium, potassium, Sulphur, magnesium and iron

Kidneys: Potassium, chlorine, fluorine, calcium, magnesium, manganese, iron, silicon

Spleen: Iron, copper, sodium, potassium, magnesium, fluorine

Lungs: Phosphorus, manganese and silicon

Gastrointestinal Tract: Sodium, potassium, calcium, chlorine, fluorine, iodine and iron

Anus: Silicon (Silicon Valley)

Bladder: Silicon and fluorine

Eyes: Sulphur and fluorine

Inner Ear: Magnesium, chlorine, fluorine, iron

Pineal Gland: Iodine, phosphorus, manganese and Sulphur

Pituitary Gland: Iodine, phosphorus, manganese, Sulphur and bromine

Adrenal Medulla: Phosphorus, Sulphur, magnesium and iodine
Adrenal Cortex: Calcium, fluorine, silicon and iron
Thyroid and Parathyroid: Sodium, potassium, magnesium, chlorine, iodine
Pancreas: Zinc, potassium, chromium and manganese
Prostate: Zinc, magnesium and silicon
Testes/Ovaries: Silicon, phosphorus, magnesium, manganese and zinc

WHAT DO THESE ELEMENTS DO?

Use this after determining what deficiencies might be existing in your body or your patient's body and how you might correct these deficiencies through the use of foods.

Oxygen: "The Healer." Every cell in your body needs oxygen Used for building, energizing, healing and burning up waste.
<u>Deficiency symptoms</u>: poor thought or memory, poor metabolism, low energy, forgetfulness, shortness of breath.
<u>High oxygen foods</u>: Liquid Chlorophyll, iron tonics, grapes, beets, tomatoes, onions, meats and wild cherries.

Carbon: The element of growth, known as "The Builder." Carbon and oxygen working together make heat.
<u>Excess symptoms are</u>: Obesity, boils, anemia, high blood pressure.
<u>To counter these problems, avoid</u>: starches, sweets, fats, meats, oily fish, fatty sausage and gravies.

Hydrogen: "The Moisturizer." Hydrogen means "water generator." Essential for blood flow, nutrient transportation, digestion, assimilation, nutrition and elimination.
<u>Deficiency symptoms</u>: Dehydration, wrinkling skin, poor bowel elimination, craving salty food, dry skin and throat, irritability, gout, arthritis, excessive body heat.

<u>Excess symptoms</u>: Puffiness under skin, loose flesh, swelling ankles, enlarged vital organs, susceptibility to heat and light.
<u>Foods high in Hydrogen</u>: Water, fruit and vegetable juices, asparagus, apricots, broccoli, mangos, melons, spinach, goat whey, cow whey, pineapples, parsley, tomatoes, sauerkraut, squash.

Calcium: Element known as "The Knitter." Calcium heals wounds, gives endurance and vitality. It buffers acid, body toning, builds and maintains the bone structure and teeth.
<u>Deficiency symptoms</u>: Lack of strength, cramps in calves, bone softening, digestive problems, abscesses, excess hemorrhaging, lack of willpower, fearful and indecisive, hungers for love, affection, sympathy, gratitude, acidic pH constitution.
<u>Excess symptoms</u>: Blunt, hard, slow, gout and growths, problems with eyes, ears and tendons.
<u>High calcium foods</u>: Kelp, cheeses, raw milks, sesame seeds, all greens, bone-broth, lemons, cottage cheese, fish, egg-yolk, cauliflower, cabbage, kale, celery, dulse.

Nitrogen: Known as "The Restrainer." It balance the explosive, radical qualities of oxygen. Nitrogen makes up about four-fifths of the atmosphere we breathe. If nitrogen were to replace oxygen in the air, breathing would subside, and death would be instantaneous. On the other hand, if nitrogen were removed, all living forms of life would burn up. Oxygen is very volatile, while nitrogen is very passive. Nitrogen keeps oxygen in place. Essential for complete metabolism, builds tissue and vitality.
<u>Excess nitrogen symptoms</u>: Romanticism, passiveness, lively imagination, mysterious, fondness for evening, nighttime, nostalgic, fleshiness, deficient immune system, susceptibility to disease.
<u>Deficiency symptoms</u>: Brain weakness, sexual weakness, feeble, numbness, muscular exhaustion, absentminded, hypochondriac, lazy and lacking desire to exert one's self.
<u>High Nitrogen foods</u>: High protein foods, fish, spices, pastas,

cheeses, nuts and seeds.

Phosphorus: The "Light Bearer" symbol of intelligence.
Phosphorus stimulates the intellect, improves nerve nutrition,
stimulates sexual functions, affects muscle tissue, acts on bone
and brain. It is present in our white blood cells. We need two
kind of phosphorus, vegetable phosphorus to feed the bones and
animal phosphorus to feed the brain. **This does not mean
vegetarians are stupid!**
Excess symptoms: Overly mental oriented, volatile emotions,
tissue degeneration, excessive confidence, vivid imagination
Deficiency symptoms: Lack of confidence, sensitive to noise,
sensitive to criticism, numbness, neuralgia, constant weakness,
fatigue.
High phosphorus foods: *Brain phosphorus foods*-Meat, egg yolk,
fish and dairy products.
Bone phosphorus foods: Almonds, soybeans, lentils, sunflower
seeds, brown rice syrup, rice bran, pumpkin and squash seeds,
wheat bran and wheat germ.

Chlorine: "The Cleanser" in its ability to expel waste from the
body, as well as freshens, purifies and disinfects. When you add
the chlorine element with another element, you create a chloride
compound. (sodium and chlorine = sodium/chloride, chlorine and
hydrogen= hydrochloric acid) Chlorine's other roles include:
increasing osmosis, decreases nerve pain and combats odor.
Excessive symptoms: Jerking, cramping muscles, craving for
salty foods, dryness of skin and tissues, muscular weakness,
nonconforming and unorthodox behavior, pessimistic,
melancholy, suspicious and apprehensive.
Deficiency symptoms: Depression, morbidity, glandular swelling,
poor appetite, painful urination, sluggish liver, restless and
anxious, sensation of a weighted pressure on head.
Chlorine food sources: Fish, raw goat milk, sauerkraut, seaweed,
celery and olives.
Sulphur: Called "The heating Element" for its ability to drive

impurities to the surface of the skin and producing heat within the body. Sulphur is a brain and nerve element. Sulphur promotes bile to flow, regulates brain heat, beautifies the complexion, build hair, skin and nails, stimulates egg and sperm production, stimulates and regulates the nerves.

<u>Deficiency symptoms</u>: Body dryness, jerky or fitfulness, weak-willed, worrisome, extreme temperature changes, cravings for fresh air and irritability.

<u>Excess symptoms</u>: Moodiness, intense emotions, forgetfulness, depression, inconsistency, falling sensations and dizziness.

<u>High Sulphur foods</u>: Brussel sprouts, kale, cabbage, watercress, horseradish, onions and potatoes.

Potassium: Known as "The Great Alkalizer" as it restores very rich alkaline salts into the blood. It also increases tissue alkalinity, aids in waste elimination, reduces acidity, supports muscular system, boosts recuperative powers, reduces pain and prevents sickness.

<u>Deficiency symptoms</u>: Acidity, mental illness, oversensitive to touch, low energy, fearfulness, tendency towards violence, reclusive and isolated.

<u>Excess symptoms</u>: Over-alkaline, bloating, gas, weakened nerves, loss of equilibrium, disruptive digestive system, dulled brain and exhaustion.

<u>Potassium-rich foods</u>: Olives, figs, grits, bananas, watercress, fish, kiwis, Jerusalem artichokes, rice bran and goat milk.

Sodium: "The Youthful Element" as it promotes limber, flexible, pliable and youthful joints. Sodium is an alkalizer. It helps prevent blood clotting, keeps calcium in solution, keeps potassium in balance, promotes the excretion of carbon dioxide, increases osmosis and is essential to all connective tissues, organs, body fluids, liver, pancreas and spleen.

<u>Deficiency symptoms</u>: Cracking joints, stiff tendons, arthritis, mental confusion, dry skin, dry tongue, frontal headache, delayed digestion, bloating or gas, lack of saliva, sensitive to drafts, poor

eyesight and murky complexion.

<u>Excess symptoms</u>: Extremist, keen reflexes, always in a hurry, accident-prone

<u>High Sodium foods</u>: Veal joint broth, goat milk, powdered whey, black mission figs, celery, sunflower seeds, apples, apricots, black olives, strawberries, fish and asparagus.

Fluorine: The "Anti-Resistant Element" known for its ability to resist decaying. (Not to be confused with the "inorganic" form put into the water supplies and other products) Calcium is reinforced by fluorine in preventing tooth decay, ulcerations and calcification, preserves youthfulness and protects from germs and infection. It also acts upon the skin, hair, bones, tooth enamel, tendons, spleen and the iris.

<u>Deficiency symptoms</u>: Falling out hair, swollen eyelids, clammy, puffy or scaly skin, disorganization, sadness in the mornings, difficulty thinking, crumbling teeth and bones, nervous stress, indifferent or worrisome.

<u>Excess symptoms</u>: Extreme sensuality, (Let's all get excess!) pessimistic towards evening time, motion discomfort, hallucinations, irritated membrane linings, (Maybe <u>don't</u> want to become excessive)"

<u>High Fluorine foods</u>: Raw fish, sea plants, raw black bass, raw green quince, raw goat milk.

Iron: The "Frisky Horse" element, because of its ability to attract oxygen. (Iron attracts oxygen, oxygen kills cancer.) Its also responsible for carrying oxygen to all tissues and organs. It improves circulation, digestion, elimination and respiration. It ensures vitality, optimism, will and courage.

<u>Deficiency symptoms</u>: Anemia, low oxygenation, depressed or melancholy, low potential energy in brain and nervous system, susceptible to colds, poor respiration, slowed speech pattern, low blood pressure, always cold, chronic tiredness.

<u>Excess symptoms</u>: Excessive brain pressure, excess blood pressure, heaviness of senses, lethargic and drowsiness.

<u>High Iron foods</u>: Liquid chlorophyll, dulse, kelp, black berries,

greens, dried fruits, black-strap molasses, egg yolks, black mission figs and black cherries.

Magnesium: "The Relaxer" because of its ability to relax everything from your brain to your bowels. Magnesium is an alkalizer. It calms the nerves and makes the body more flexible. It induces restful sleep, lowers fevers and cools the body, acts as a laxative and purifies the body of toxic acids, gases and impurities. Magnesium prevents phosphates from precipitating in our joints. It is said to relieve many who complain of backaches. In mental patients, in high doses, it has proven effective in restoring 80% back to a state of health.
Deficiency symptoms: Hyperactive nervous system, hot tempered, drastic mood shifts, sleeplessness, neuralgia, forgetfulness, aches and headaches.
Excess symptoms: Defective memory, slowed perceptions, incoherent speech problems, sleepiness, dulled intellect.
Foods high in Magnesium: Nuts, green, wheat germ, whole grains, berries, yellow cornmeal, soybeans, onion tops, endive, dried figs, dried bananas, apples, cabbage, cashews, beet tops, fish, goat milk, brown rice, rye, parsley, spinach, watercress and whole wheat.

Silicon: Called "The Magnetic Element" as, from out of its presence in the human body, comes a magnetic personality, charm and the beauty of movement. Silicon is responsible for the sheen and resilience of the hair, skin and nails. Nerve transmission would be impossible without silicon. Silicon acts as a link or neurotransmitter between blood and nerves. Silicon carries the nerve impulse. It also adds rigidity, firmness and toughness to bones, teeth and tendons, reinforces membranes, walls, ligaments, linings, helps retain body heat and electricity, increases strength, resistance and energy.
Excess symptoms: Overactive intelligence, optimist, cheerfulness, graceful and agile, spontaneous, good speech and finger dexterity, constantly active and overconfident.

(Sound like just the <u>right</u> amount to me.)
<u>Deficiency symptoms</u>: Hair falling out, crackling and swelling joints, weakness in the ligaments, fatigue and loss of strength, nervous stomach, low body temperature, mental strain, excessive foot perspiration, tender spine, skin abscesses, scabs and scales and alternating sleepiness to sleeplessness.
<u>High Silicon foods</u>: Brown rice syrup, rice polishings, oats, barley, nuts, kelp and cereal grains.

Iodine: Named "The Metabolizer" for its ability in regulating the metabolism. Iodine's role in the human prevents goiters, vital for thyroid, spleen and liver, neutralizes albumin, aids in assimilation of calcium, chlorine, silicon and fluorine, vital to brain function and prevents sores and ulcers. Iodine is the first element in the DNA code for brain development.
<u>Deficiency symptoms</u>: Goiter, extreme nervousness, awkwardness, childlike behavior, heart and lung problems, mental degeneration, dull ache under scapular bones, restless and rolling eyeballs, flabby, doughy skin, hyperthyroidism or hypothyroidism. One has too little iodine and the other is burning it up too fast, Either way, iodine deficiency. Iodine is an incredible anti-virus and bactericide.
<u>Excess symptom</u>: Protruding or bulging eyeballs, nervous or anxious, nerve tremors, fear of the future, acute sense of touch.
<u>Foods high in Iodine</u>: Dulse, kelp, sea plants and fish

Manganese: It is known as "The Love Element for the reason that parents deprived of this element, turn hostile toward their young. In laboratory mice, they eat their babies. Manganese is known best for its role in controlling nerves, thought and action coordinator and memory improvement. Also known to improve eyesight, taste, touch, smell and hearing.
Excess symptoms: Exaggerated emotions, intensified sensations
Deficiency symptoms: Cracking joints, gout symptoms, nightmares, impatient, anxieties, quarrelsome, mental confusion, reoccurring swollen glands, headaches for motion, reduced

appetite, reduced thirst.

Foods high in Manganese: Nuts and seeds, (Missouri black walnuts) So, everyone here in the Ozarks should have enhanced intellectual powers with coordinated thoughts and actions!

ENZYMES

This can end up being a fascinating subject when you start researching enzymes and what they actually do. They are amazing! So, on we go.

Everyone knows digestive enzymes help digest our foods. There are four basic digestive enzymes: Amylase (starches), Lipase (lipids or fats), Protease (protein) and Cellulase (plant fiber). We know they are enzymes because they end in the suffix "ase."

There are two categories of these digestive enzymes: endogenous (those produced in our bodies) and exogenous (those found in raw foods). The "endogenous" enzymes are produced mainly by our pancreas and liver. The more of the "exogenous" enzymes we consume, the less work our body has to do making enzymes and the more energy we reserve for other metabolic processes. This means our pancreas and liver are less likely to swell up from all the extra work load.

Enough with the "digestive" enzyme stuff.

Did you know: we have approximately 300,000 different enzymes in our bodies and only about 3,000 of them have been isolated and job categorized? Digestive enzymes make up only a very small fraction of total enzymes in your body.

During a day, your liver is going to produce over 4 to 5 billion enzymes. Enzymes are responsible for every process that happens with our bodies. If it weren't for enzymes, we would not be able to sustain life. What regulates our blood pressure, the heart? No, enzymes. What opens and closes the valves to our heart? Enzymes. Enzymes keep our blood pH perfect. Enzymes play a huge role in the physical attraction between man and woman. They are numerously contributing to the marvel of sexuality, and to the wonder of sex itself. Enzymes provide the energy for the sperm to travel to the ovum, and upon contact, another enzyme opens the door of the ovum, allowing the sperm to enter, and yet another enzyme closes the door as to let no other intruders into the egg. Enzymes are the soldiers that come out to put our wounds back together. Enzymes help to build new tissues and cells as we need them, remove metabolic waste from our systems and play a huge role in our immune system. We have enzymes for thinking, enzymes for laughing. We even have an enzyme that stops us from crying, and if it were not present, we would actually continue crying until dehydration. Ever watch lightening bugs flashing around on a hot summer night and wonder how that light works? Its because of an enzyme called "Luciferase."

Within the nucleus of each of our cells are 23 chromosomes from our mother and another 23 from our father. Together, these program a blend of all the family traits, or "genes" passed down through the "gene"-rations and the unique expression of our individuality. Our DNA molecules are programmed through these chromosome genes, making this the actual memory of the cell. Within each individual cell there are roughly 100,000 genes and guess what, the majority of these genes are encoded for specific enzyme functions. With approximately 75 trillion cells, each with 100,000 genes…well, that's a lotta genes! Most of which are programmed for enzyme activity. We are a world of enzymes. To put it in the words of D.A. Lopez, M.D. *"Within the sum total of our bodies, enzymes work constantly like a majestic orchestra conducting a splendid symphony in perfect harmony."* It could not have been put more gloriously profound. There is a wonderous adventure in the tiny micro-universe of enzymes. I suggest you continue to research and discover your own amazing worlds.

I'm not going to spend anymore time on this subject. But there are many wonderful books out there on these enzymes. If you are interested in further research, may I suggest: Food enzymes, The Missing Link to Radiant Health, by Humbart Santillo. This is a good beginner's book for understanding digestive enzymes.

A more technical, but fascinating book on all enzymes and

their mechanical functions in the human body is:

"Enzymes, The Fountain of Life," by D.A. Lopez, R.M. Williams and M. Miehlke.

CHAPTER 5

WHY DO WE NEED WATER?

Your body is 70-80 percent water. All body chemistry reactions take place in water. Water is the first most important requirement for the liver to function properly. Water is the key to all bodily functions. Water is responsible for and involved in nearly every bodily process, including digestion, absorption, circulation and elimination. Water is the primary transporter of nutrients throughout the body. Your brain is 75% water, your Heart 75%, Lungs and Liver both 85%, Kidneys 83%, Muscles 75% and your blood is 83% water. Water is essential for carrying metabolic wastes from the body as well as helping in regulating body temperature.

Our blood is 94% of the total body's water supply. If that supply is low, our 94% is also low. This means our vessels shrink to take up the extra left-over room, leading to a major cause of high blood pressure. NOT a deficiency in blood pressure meds.

We must have water for cellular function. Water is a hydroelectric generator. It creates voltage. It also transfers nutrients in and toxins out of our cells.

Frequent headaches or leg cramps can be the first signs of dehydration.

Asthma, Heartburn, dyspepsia, Rheumatoid joint pains, migraine headaches and Bulimia are just a few more illnesses triggered by dehydration.

Thirst is an indicative sign that the body is already in dehydration. When we continually deprive the body of water, the body will evolve into the illusion that water is unavailable, and the thirst mechanism will be shut off. Now, we'll never know when we're thirsty. Interesting thing about that is, and I suffer from this same plague, a pregnant mother not drinking enough water and remaining in a dehydration state will pass the thirst shut-off state on to their baby. My mother NEVER drank water and would wake up in the mornings unable to speak because her mouth was basically dried out clear down her throat. Every illness she battled, including the one that took her life, were water dehydration related.

WHAT'S THE BEST WATER TO DRINK?

I am not going to answer that question, as this is as varied of an opinionated subject as soy, coconut oil, politics and religion.. What I am going to do is give you facts and characteristics of various water types and let you form your own opinion, if you have not already.

There are different waters and different needs of each individual. Some waters will be wetter water, some higher mineral content, some more alkaline, etc. I will give you the information and let you determine which is best for you.

Let's start off with distilled water, as it is the most controversial and also the purest of water, having all its minerals removed, leaving more room for water molecules

.

DISTILLED WATER- is considered by some, to be the superior water and by others, to be the worst of choice. But here are the facts.

The highest energy water comes from the steam distillation process. No other water type is able to transport minerals into the system as steam distilled water.

Nature, our tutor, uses the distillation water process first, through evaporation, then returning the distilled water to earth as rain. If distilled water were not the finest form, nature would not be using it predominately. Animals will most always choose distilled water over any other. There are two forms of natural distilled water: rain water and glacier water. This glacier water is one of the reasons the people of the Hunza Valley regard it as being responsible for their rate of 129 to 150 years of age.

I know, we have all heard the horror stories of how distilled water leeches all your minerals from your body. Have you ever seen a piece of your liver floating in the toilet, or a piece of a kidney, or even a bone? The minerals have already been incorporated into your body parts. For the water to flush the minerals out of our body, it would have to be flushing out parts of our organs. There are free floating minerals in body fluids they may be flushed, but that is true with any water or liquid if you are not adequately replenishing the mineral supply.

Your body must distill ALL water before it can be utilized by the body. The liver has to put water on the body's frequency, like all other types of food. High energy water is much easier to convert than low energy water. All other mineral waters, hard, or soft, are considered "light water The mineral in hard water has taken the energy away from the water molecule making it low in energy. It is also a dryer water. Wet water is soft, high in energy, low in minerals and "heavy. (not to be confused with "Heavy Water or deuterium.) Light waters are hard, high mineral, dryer and low energy. Steam distilled water adds energy. Here are the characteristics of distilled water:

1. Contains no minerals therefore, there is no conflict with attached electrical frequencies and no minerals of the type for the body to use. This is a very important factor when we are working on adjusting frequencies or tweaking the liver voltage.
2. Wetter water, no minerals, allowing for more water molecules per surface area.
3. Having no minerals, there is no problem of out-of-solution minerals interfering with bodily functions. Ever seen lyme deposits accumulate of your faucets? That's what can also happen to your joints, muscles and tissues when improper forms of minerals are present.
4. There is much less surface tension in distilled water, meaning the water creates a higher conductivity at the cellular level. This in addition to smaller water molecules, makes it more permeable and easier to pass into and out of your cells..
5. Distilled water is the preferred water during cleanses. Also by Nature.

There is one more contradiction I would like to clear up. There is a myth going around on the internet that distilled water is "acidic." This is simply not true. I have personally tested sample after sample of steam distilled water with a very expensive pH meter and I have yet to find one sample registering less than 7.0 pH which is neutral. Many tested in the alkaline range. Distilled water is wonderful for gout, arthritis and rheumatism. Joint deposits, toxins, gases and inorganic minerals are dissolved and flushed out with distilled water.

Its true, a water containing no minerals cannot replenish your mineral supply. However, if you are eating healthy you should be acquiring these minerals through your food sources. But distilled water will not leech your minerals out of your bones and organs, as they have become already incorporated into those areas.

Let's examine and compare the other popular types of water. Since we have already started with what Mother Nature considers the optimal form, we will continue from that direction to the worst.

REVERSE OSMOSIS- This is the next in line to distilled water. It is a process of charcoal filtration and is the only way besides distilling to remove the TDS (Total Dissolved Solvents) which includes heavy metals, toxins and pesticides that have been absorbed through the ground and into the water supply. You can find TDS meters on Amazon, Ebay and even at Wal-Mart for around ten bucks and test your own water in about ten seconds.

BOTTLED SPRING WATER- IF you are unable to access the first two water types, this would be your next choice. However, there are varying degrees of purity in these waters, depending on the cleanliness, filtration system and the company's over-all concern with the health of the consumer. I personally know a very popular brand sold nationwide that actually fills their bottles up from a hose with absolutely no processing or filtration system, whatsoever and this is bottled as "purified spring water." Then, there's the plastic.

WELL WATER- Well water is still one step and can be several steps above city tap water. Well water contains a high amount of TDS that need to be filtered out, which can be removed through reverse osmosis. In addition to the TDS's, well water also contains parasites that have not been exterminated, unless you treat the well with toxic chemicals such as chlorine, which just turned it into an undesirable water source and in need of R.O.. The natural, safe and healthy way to rid the well water of parasites would be installing an ultraviolet light on the water system that creates ozone. This would assure the death of these little critters. Then, of course, you would still want to filter the water after the ozone machine as to not be ingesting millions of DEAD microscopic corpses.

SOFT WATER- This type of water should not be consumed unless it has been filtered through reverse osmosis or at least a three-stage micro-screening filtration system. Then, it is not entirely unacceptable. This water softener sodium can very hard on the human body. (some may disagree) While there have been no conclusive studies to the actual detriments of water softener water, we are warned not to water our lawn and plants with the stuff. I opt, for that reason alone, not to water my body with softened water.

TAP WATER- Tap water, bar none, is the worst water you can ingest into your body, with the exception of radioactive waste runoff or contaminated swamp water. Besides the chlorine and fluoride in the water, the minerals in most water, especially tap water, are in the wrong form for our bodies to use.

We have all seen the calcium that gather on our faucets from "hard water." This is precisely what they will do inside your body when they are not of the correct organic form. They will precipitate in your joints, arteries, your liver and other organs. The term "hard water" is very correct in the context that it is very hard on your system.

We understand now that ALL elements have an electrical frequency attached. We also know that we are constantly adjusting our frequencies when we are consuming these elements. Nine times out of ten, the frequencies attached to the metals and minerals found in these waters are not of the proper frequencies we are looking for and will thus work against our balancing progress.

However, the TDS of most tap water has been reduced to what the government classifies as healthy, if that is of any consolation. But, this water still remains at the bottom of the list.
The World Health Organization considers water with 300 mg/liter acceptable to drink. While that may be acceptable, is it healthy? That's 300 milligrams per liter of anything from metals

to medicine to toxic fertilizers and insecticides. My personal standard is below 30. If you are worried about minerals lacking, take a supplement and eat as I am showing you in this book. You will have ample minerals in your system and will be far outperforming these government officials that are sliding by with the least amount of quality possible.

SPECIALTY WATERS- Nowadays, we have all these eccentric and exotic waters: High Alkaline Water, Smart Water, High Mineral Water, Charged Ionic Water, Molecular Memory Locked Waters, etc. These are , of varying degrees, fairly acceptable waters. Some are fun, some are fantastic, and some are gimmick waters. Of course, as with everything, you must read the labels and do some research. Some contain high amounts of sugar, some have high sodium and others contain various undesirable ingredients and additives.

ARE YOU PROGRAMMED BY YOUR ENVIRONMENT?

If someone pulled a gun on you, would you not assume that person has intent to harm you? If a dog is barreling at you, growling, steam puffing out his nostrils, saliva spraying all over his face and his teeth snapping like a Mako shark, would you not begin to get the idea he's not coming over for a belly rub and now might be a good time to start planning a quick exit strategy 'cause you're about to become dog lunch?

In both of these instances, you perceived danger. Your eyes received the image and sent it to your brain for processing. Your brain then perceived the situation as harmful or dangerous. Just as with every thought, this perception is then forwarded to every cell in your body. Your cells have been "Enviro-stimulated," programmed by an outside stimuli that was first initiated through the only link between the outside world around you and the world inside you, your eyes or "your preceptors."

What makes a shy person shy? What makes a defensive person defensive? Where does the personality trait develop? Where does it come from? What makes a person frightened all the time? What makes a child consistently lash out in anger for no apparent reason? What makes any of what we are? Of course , our life experiences play a large role in creating the person we become. But, what about children? What about newborns? I'm going to take you on a journey into a fascinating a relative new world of discovery, the science of Quantum Physics. This small-particle world was not even known to exist until fairly recently. Now, it has opened the doors, eyes and minds of scientists and enthusiasts throughout the world. It is teaching us, in many ways, how the universe and Nature interact.

Long, long ago, in a dark and liquid world, far different than the illuminated ether and oxygen world you exist in at present, you were being programmed of emotional and personality traits. Most of us have been led to believe our personalities are adaptations that are molded and sculpted after birth from our life's experiences, or in other words, "products of our environment." This is only a partially correct truism. While still encapsulated within your mother's womb, before you were able to make decisions on your own, before you were fully developed, before you could talk, or even breathe, through enviro-stimulation, you were being genetically encoded to ascertain certain characteristics.

Your "preceptors," your eyes, your link to the outside world, had not fully developed, nor could they function within this darkened, liquid environment. So, you had to rely on other means of connecting to this outer world in which you had not yet arrived or experienced. That connection was your mother's eyes. These preceptors were your means of exploring this undiscovered world. The mother's eyes, seemingly quite disconnected from and incapable of any response to the unborn child, actually are very connected and play quite an incredible role in the developing personality of the unborn child.

If you have outstanding traits, be they good or bad, you may want to examine your world before birth. You may just uncover some very interesting characteristics or influential events that may have occurred during your gestation period.

This example is from an Italian film clip during an experiment, using ultra-sonic photography on a pregnant woman's womb, to prove any possibilities of supporting this theory. You will find this very enlightening and it WILL stimulate you to see things from a different perspective. It might even throw caution to the wind on how you want to act around your unborn baby.

As the film clip goes, an ultrasound of a baby laying in the mother's womb, is resting quietly in its single occupancy, seemingly safe environment. When suddenly, the silence is shattered with the shouting of an angry male voice. Simultaneously, with the first shout, the fetus responds by jumping several inches in the womb. Instantly, is heard a crash, such as that of a heavy book being thrown upon a desk or a table. Again, the noise is immediately responded as the unborn again leaps several inches off its peaceful resting place in this presumably, safe environment.

This is the eyewitness example of "enviro-stimulation." What has just occurred here and how does this apply to us in any way, shape or form? The mother has just perceived, through her eyes or her "preceptors," which transmitted the perception to her "receptor" (her brain) that this is a hostile environment. That thought, just as it passes through every cell in her body, via the bloodstream, through the placenta and into the baby. What then, has just occurred? The unborn, perceiving through the mother's eyes, via the placenta, receives a warning that it is about to enter a hostile or dangerous environment.

So, what happens next? The baby comes out, and from the forewarning, responds by being either a frightened child, clinging to mother for constant protection, or it is a very defensive child, always trying to push everything and everyone away to stay out of danger.

You see, the mother, having a screaming and possibly abusive partner, perceived her environment as being dangerous and hostile. The impression was relayed to her unborn baby to, "prepare and fend for yourself. You are about to enter a much more dangerous situation" and, "Voila," both the mother and father, with no knowledge of the fact, have in essence, been genetically engineering their unborn child through an unseen channel at the quantum or small particle level.

This is the science behind playing soothing music or reading to the unborn. The vibrational frequencies of the music can be just as effective without the music going first, through the auditory preceptors, the ears, of the mother, before being transferring to the fetus.

Ever wonder why a mother 500 miles away, can sense danger with one of her children? We must turn to quantum physics for that answer. First let us establish the fact, energy can't be destroyed. You can crush an atom, but it only becomes smaller particles and replicas of the whole. Here is the key: If you split an atom in half, take one of the halves five hundred miles away, hit the other half with an electrical charge, the first half will jump simultaneously. Though the umbilical cord has been severed on the physical plane, in the quantum world, it remains attached. The mother and child will share this connection forever, even beyond the physical world. It can never be destroyed. It's a fascinating and magical world, isn't it?

CHAPTER 6

EATING FOR A HEALTHY BODY AND SOUL

Eating when upset is definitely a bad time to be putting food in your mouth. When you are stressed, your adrenal glands are opened up which means your digestive system is pretty much shut down. Your food will still go down the pipe and it will get processed, to a degree, at least enough for elimination. But the chance of any significant nutrient extraction and nutritional absorption is unlikely. The digestion process takes so much energy, the other systems are shutting down to conserve more energy to devote to the digestive process. However, when the adrenal glands are activated, the digestive system is also shut down.

The adrenals are our "Fight or Flight" glands. They are all about protection. They are all about "kick butt" or run like hell to save ours! When the adrenals are energized, whether from fear, anger, sadness or just plain stressed out, they have no way of knowing the difference. All they know is they have been activated, so all systems must be conserved to prepare for defensive tactics. The immune system is shut down to a minimal, as well as is digestion.

While the adrenals are putting out the amber alert to cut back all systems, without the incredible amount of energy needed for the digestive process to be completed, the job just cannot be executed adequately. The adrenals are about the only entity in your body that takes precedence over the digestive process. That makes them pretty powerful. Look at them like our "Secretary of Defense."

Eating when we're relaxed, not being rushed, having a good time and being able to savor and enjoy the food we're putting in our mouth is the best time to eat. Obviously, that's not always a feasible or available choice in this day and age, or is it?

We all seem compelled to push our lives faster and faster, like being in a revolving door that we keep pushing faster and faster until we can't keep up with the newly created centrifuge, and we surely can't slow down because the weight and centrifugal force of this vortex forces us to keep up or be squished. Slow down a bit. Take a "time out." At least long enough to have a relaxing meal. We all have bills to pay, but no need to turn them into doctor bills.

As you are eating, how many of us, while we are still chewing, are already stabbing into our food, loading up our fork for that next bite? Do we even taste the food that's already in our mouth? How well are we chewing this food? We do this, not because of fish bones, as Lucille Ball would have you believe, but to help take some of the work load off the digestive system.

Chewing is the first stage of digestion. It not only breaks down the food particles, but in the saliva is an enzyme called "ptyalin," an Amylase enzyme, which is the first stage of carbohydrate digestion. This is why it is so important to chew our food into a liquid state or "chyme" and mix it well with the saliva. You also will savor each bite more thoroughly, enjoy the taste of what you're eating, the food will last longer and best of all, you will end up not eating as much. Your "full" mechanism will actually have a chance to register and tell you its time to stop, instead of shoving it all in so fast the only reason you know you're done is because you've run out of food. THERE'S NOTHING ELSE LEFT TO SHOVE IN! Besides, when your boss asks why you're back late from lunch? Health reasons! You won't be lying. Send me a self-addressed, stamped envelope and I'll mail you a doctor's excuse to take longer lunches. Chew your food and enjoy it. Life will taste better, and you will enjoy it longer.

THE DEATH KRONE'S DIET

*"One should look where one is going,
                or one is likely to end up where one is headed."*
                Old Chinese proverb

Many people think they are cooking and eating to live, when in essence, they are cooking and eating to die.

One third of what we eat keeps us alive, the other two thirds keep the doctor alive. Man creates either health or disease at the table. Disease, by eating foods that have been overcooked, processed beyond the point of any nutritional value, genetically altered and loaded with chemicals, preservatives, food coloring, hydrogenated oils and DEATH.

Don't think because you haven't had any trips to the hospital for by-pass surgery and you haven't had your gallbladder taken out or your appendix removed, that it can't or won't happen. Keep walking that tight-wire. Keep over-consuming greasy, fried foods, excessive dairy, too much meat, wheat, sodas, processed sugar-ladened deserts, caffeine, preservatives and all the other comfort foods the FDA labels as fit for human consumption, because you will end up "<u>gravely</u>" mistaken. Knock on the door of the Death Krone enough times and sooner or later, someone will answer.

"END" DIGESTION

Its seems its becoming a fad to be ill these days. In fact, with the barrage of T.V. ads for medicines and hospitals, it makes you feel like you're not normal if you're healthy. Just look at all these new medical procedures and medicines they're discovering. Look at all the great questions they've come up with, just for you, so you can ask your doctor. And you're sitting there missing out on all this great stuff just because "you're healthy."

Why do so many Americans suffer from "heartburn" or acid indigestion? Is it because they're deficient in one or more of the inorganic chemicals that lay inside the "Purple Pill?" No. *"Ask your doctor if the purple pill is right for you."* Go ahead, ask him. Ten to one odds he'll say, "yes, it is." And write you out a prescription for a symptom suppressor that you may be on the rest of your life and possibly destroys your liver

.

Want to know the main causes of heartburn or acid reflux?
#1-Lack of Hydrochloric acid. This is made from 1 molecule of hydrogen and 1 molecule of chlorine. Most people are deficient in the chlorine from lack of eating enough chlorine foods like, Brussel sprouts, broccoli, asparagus, fish, goat milk, not because they're old and can't make it.
#2- Digestive enzymes are weak from liver pH being out of ideal range. Food ferments instead of digests.

Could you imagine if your doctor told you to go to the store,

62

buy yourself some organic fruits and vegetables, cut your acid consumption down, adjust your pH's, take some Betaine HCL and your heartburn and acid-reflux will go away? Not much money to be made by <u>solving</u> the problem.

I have another question: If your doctor DID tell you to do all of these things, would you? You CAN get to the root of this problem and do away with it completely and forever. Let's investigate just how to go about doing just that.

First of all, let's break the main food down into….awwwh, you didn't think I was just going to tell you what to take and be done with it? No, I want you to know exactly how it works, so it makes total sense and you can explain it to others.

So, we're breaking our food down into two food categories which are going to be Proteins and Starches/Carbohydrates. Protein needs acidic digestive environment and the starches and carbs are combined because both need alkalinity to digest.

When we eat starches, we must first "chew our food well" mixing it with as much saliva as possible, as the first stage of carb digestion takes place in the mouth, as I mentioned before. From this point on, until the food reaches the colon ready for evacuation, the digestive process takes place in a totally "alkaline" environment. (above 7.0 pH)

Not so, for protein digestion. As the protein food enters the stomach, hydrochloric acid or HCL is released creating a very acidic environment, as the HCL is needed to break down the protein capsules. After the protein exits the stomach, it enters the small intestine. From there to the colon, the remaining digestive process is totally alkaline, same as with the carbohydrates.

Theoretically, if we could by-pass the stomach process, we could mix the protein with the starches and they would be totally compatible. However, (you knew that was coming) this is not the case. When we introduce protein, acidic fruit, acidic beverages or any other acid-forming substance during the totally needed alkaline environment of the carbohydrate digestion process, we initially stop the digestive process of the carbohydrate altogether, dead in its tracks. This leads to carbohydrate fermentation, which leads to gas, bloating, a very acidic state and "End-Digestion."

The inherited American diet goes something like this:

Breakfast: Eggs, ham, toast, or biscuits, hash-browns and coffee.
        (acid)(acid)(acid)   (acid)   (acid)   (acid)
Lunch: Quarter-pounder, fries and soda or tea
         (acid)   (acid) (acid) (acid)
Dinner: Meat and potatoes, green beans, bread and coffee
    (acid)   (acid)   (alkaline) (acid)   (acid)

Let's start with the breakfast. We had eggs, ham and coffee, all being acid-forming. Then, we added bread and potatoes, which are carbs and starches. So, now we have created a fermentation situation, "End-Digestion." We mixed carbs with the protein. The carbs had to be alkaline while the proteins need acid digestion environment. We could have left out the bread.

Now, for lunch we had again, ALL acidic foods. No fermentation there. But wait a minute…wasn't there bread on the Quarter Pounder? Uh, oh…"End-Digestion."

Time for dinner. Oh, good, we have an "All-American" combination of meat protein and starch, "End-Digestion." Then, let's wash it all down with a cup of black "acid-reflux."
All done? Let's go lay down so this stuff can digest. Sorry, it probably won't. It will lie there, (with you) fermenting, causing gas pains, belching, acid-reflux, all-round discomfort and "End-Di….wait for it…gestion." No nutritional absorption, and how much electricity did we produce? "Honey, go get me the Tums! Forget that, bring me a "Purple Pill!" Add to that a side of "Liver Transplant."

THE PERFECT MEAL?

We have a young friend going through her first year of schooling to be an R.N.. Over lunch, she recently shared with us the perfect meal, as taught by a "board certified" dietitian on the nutritional end of the training. We were appalled when she revealed "Le Pesisto Plat du'jour." That perfect meal was none other than: a quarter-pounder with cheese, fries and a coke. Are these people out of their freakin' minds? The lettuce and tomato are the ONLY thing remotely resembling anything that should even be eaten. And you can be quite certain they are not organic and I'm pretty sure NOT Non-GMO.

The bread: bleached, white flour, water and yeast (glue). Completely empty calories, devoid of any nutrition what-so-ever. This is the stuff to glue your intestinal tract shut, while at the same time, promoting food allergies and celiac disease. And let's talk "End-Digestion."

The burger: A dead piece of meat someone tried to pass off as a cow. This, according to all research reports, is some of the lowest grade meat one could expect to find (or hope never to find). It is ladened with growth hormones, steroids, antibiotics and preservatives. You can keep it for over a year, and it will look as good as it did the day you bought it. It will taste about the same as well. Try it! Then its cooked in pure, saturated fat and just waiting for that colonoscopy to be ordered. Confucius say, "Better to put roots down mouth, than rod up butt!" Now, I don't know if Confucius really said that. It might have just been my twisted sense of humor.

The cheese: is made from the over-heated stuff that turns into something very similar to plastic, creating plastic cellular membranes, nothing goes in and nothing comes out. It is mucous-forming, mold, yeast and fungus-ladened and the poorest of what the FDA calls food grade, cheap, "not-cheese.

Let's look at the thing that once used to be a potato: greasy, trans-fat, artery-clogging, free-radical, nutrition-less garbage.

Soda- We won't even insult our own intelligence by pretending there could be the remotest possibility of finding the slightest of anything healthy or nutritious in the soda. Its twice as acidic as a dead cell, eats battery acid, pumps your sugar beyond high and stacks fat cell after fat cell on your belly, your butt and anywhere else it can find to cling.

These are "Board Certified Nutritionists" that are supposed to know what they're talking about. I've seen people wheeled into their room after just having had heart by-pass surgery and the first meal to build their health back, the first meal served is: fried bacon, fried eggs, sausage, white toast, a pot of coffee and a salt shaker. What's wrong with this picture? What's wrong with our logic? What caused us to need by-pass surgery in the first place? It sure wasn't organic fruits and vegetables. Now, that doesn't bother some people out there because this standard has been accepted. Hey, its "FDA approved." It has to be healthy! It bothers me!

Let's add it all up and see just what kind of nutritional benefits and wonderful health side effects we've created with this "perfect meal."

We've ingested a meat that will lay in our digestive tract for approximately five years, pumped our bodies full of steroids, growth hormones, anti-biotics, trans-fats, cholesterol, added to the already over-consumption of glue-forming, colon-clogging bleached-white flour that eventually glues our colon shut, added more mold, yeast and fungus to our system with a side of carcinogenic preservatives and pure stick-it-to-your-ribs, hang-it-from-your-gut, slap-it-on-yer-butt, FAT. Then, we wash it all down with a glass of A.D.D. sugar-ladened acid wash. Now, that's a meal!

Oh, wait! I almost forgot the slice of pesticided, half-ripened **tomato** and the leaf of nutrient-free, preserved Round-Up head-lettuce with probably food coloring and nitrates or nitrites to keep it looking fresh.

These last two items were the only thing that had a chance of actually making it to the list of healthy items. But they have been shot down and degraded with proven carcinogenic chemicals. Even the mustard and ketchup are fermented, food colored and preserved. Nothing more than mold, yeast and fungus cultivators. But it all tastes good and that's what counts, isn't it?

I can't imagine anyone over-looking this absolutely perfect meal. Its got it all! For one cheap price, you get your arteries clogged, blood pressure raised, big dose of blubber, food allergens, hormone stimulation, free-radicals, arterial wall deterioration, mold, yeast, fungus, colon glued, constipation, indigestion and a good shot of carcinogens and total acid saturation.

Why wouldn't anyone consider this to be the perfect meal? Just think, if you just keep eating this perfect meal day-after-day-after-day, with all that non-digestible meat and glue, you too can soon be walking around with your prolapsed colon dangling around your knees. Or better yet, going to the toilet in that bag hanging around your waist. It's the perfect American meal, FDA approved and all. And to top it all off, I bet your doctor has a pill for that.

I want to make perfectly clear. I am not saying McDonalds is trying to deliberately poison people with their food. They definitely provide meals for a very low price. I am not saying, don't eat at McDonalds. But, let's get real here people. The perfect meal, it is NOT. Not from a health standpoint, anyway.

Its time to wake up, step up and take responsibility for our health and longevity. No more excuses; "Well, I'm just always in such a hurry." "My boss wouldn't understand." "I don't know what to fix." "I don't know how to fix it." "I don't have a way to store it at work." "People will make fun of me." Yea, well slow down, make him understand, learn how, find a way and become a leader and not the guest of honor at the visitation service.

Forget the convenience. Forget the simplicity. Forget the speed. If you don't, the only thing that truly matters, you're speeding towards your own death.

So, how do I eat, now that I have learned I can't mix meat with anything and I can't drink anything before, during or after meals, and fruits and vegetables can't be mixed with anything and my favorite happy meal can't making me happy anymore?

Its really not all that bad. Here's a simplified version of the rules of eating and food combining.

1. **Never mix Beef and Bread** (Protein and carbohydrates) need different pH environment to digest. Never a good combination. "But what about my ham sandwich, or my Quarter Pounder?" Sorry.
2. **Eat Fruit Alone**. They are quick digesting and need alkalinity will be less likely to ferment. However, they can be eaten with green, leafy vegetables that are high in water content. To eat fruit alone is to avoid digestive disaster like gas and bloating from fermentation.
3. **Eat Protein with Non-Starchy Vegetables**. They both need

an acidic environment to digest. Non-starchy vegetables have enough intact enzymes to digest themselves without the need for and an alkaline environment, as long as they have not been overcooked as to destroy the enzymes.

4. **Eat Starches with Healthy Fats and Vegetables.** Starches (such as bread, pasta, brown rice, cous-cous and quinoa), along with starchy vegetables (such as sweet potatoes, peas, corn and squash), need an alkaline environment for digestion. This is the reason, starches combine best when eaten together.

5. **Leafy Greens and Non-Starchy Veggies mix with All Foods** Again, foods come equipped with their own enzymes and not in need of the alkaline environment.

6. **Drink one glass of water** 30 minutes before meal and 1 ½ hours after. Water is important to help break down foods but be careful as to drinking too close to eating, as this will dilute your digestive enzymes. It is also best not to drink ice cold water, as the heat needed for digestion may be hindered with the drop in temperature.

7. **Spice and Herbs** are wonderful, as they are considered neutral.

8. **Beans and Legumes** are a harder food to place in a food combining category, as they are both a protein and a starch. But, as they are primarily considered a starch, it is best to kept them paired with vegetables and other starches.

Now, before you run off saying, "This guy's outta his friggin' mind, taken away my bologna sandwich, my bacon and sodies," let me say this: You can keep eating the same habitual ways you are accustomed to. Its not going to kill you or anything like that, yet. These are merely tips and suggestions for better nutritional absorption, easier digestion and less discomfort. Did you know that lab tests show the carbohydrates in most persons are 80% still intact. In other words, the carbohydrates found in examined fecal matter, are only 20 percent digested. This is the result of poor food combining, the result of adding protein or acidic drinks to a carbohydrate alkaline digestive process.

If you eat a bagel, which needs an alkaline environment, and you are in the midst of chewing up your third bite of this bagel, and you decide to wash it down with one swallow of coffee, you just ended the digestive process of that bagel, totally and forever. Its comin' out the other end nearly as intact as when it went in the first end. Only difference being, you chewed on it first. So, when we fail to take the time to separate our food combinations, we lose much of our valuable nutrition. We might have satisfied our taste buds but what have we done for the nutritional needs of our cells and our organs? Have we satisfied their taste buds?

And now, the next obstacle to overcome.....

BUT WHAT DO I SAY TO MY CHILDREN?

Young people think they are immune to the abuse they are continually subjecting their bodies to; fast foods, burgers, hot dogs, fried this, fried that, sodas, alcohol, processed sugars, preservatives, food coloring, energy drinks, cigarettes, vapes, etc. Parents think they are being "good" parents when they give their children a treat of candy or ice-cream and "bad" parents when they limit or remove the consumption of these health-degenerative foods. They cleaned their room so, treat them with some candy and cavities? They took a nap so, give them ice-cream, a stomach-ache, attention deficit disorder, poor heath and possible diabetes? Thanks, Mom! Thanks, Dad!

When it comes to small children, they are at our mercy. We must learn to keep them healthy. We must form their life-long habits as good healthy ones, so they may continue to stay healthy. It is proven that what a child learns in his first seven years, sticks. Teach them while they're young. Then, teach the grandparents and aunts and uncles that they must, under no circumstances, go against your decisions.

Forget what Sally's mother puts in her child's lunch. Forget what Bobby's parents might think because you've instructed them not to feed processed sugars and fried foods to your child when he or she visits their house for dinner. Tell the aunts, uncles, grandparents and anyone else that may have an opportunity to feed your child, exactly what they are allowed and not allowed to eat. Then, so you won't sound like a crazed, dominating, paranoid control-freak-a-zoid, lunatic, explain to them, why. They may absorb a morsel or two of knowledge themselves. And who knows, you may have just started the beginning of saving a whole lot of lives. Don't be afraid to take charge. Is an "image" worth as much as your child's health?

Jimmy has a cough and a cold all of the time. Suzie has asthma. Lilly, has to have allergy shots every week. Jack has A.D.D. (attention deficit disorder) and is failing his classes. Every time Amie turns around, she gets the flu. Jimmy, Suzie and Lillie ALL drink way too much milk, eat way too much dairy and wheat products. Jack is toxic and allowed to eat too many foods containing processed sugar. He's wired. Amie, is also toxic and her immune system fragile and unable to fend for itself.

Most of the kids are sick nowadays, most of the time. Why? Not because there's a germ-fest marathon, its because their bodies are toxic, out of balance and their immune systems are weak from improper nutrition, lack of and foods made from nutritionally valueless junk.

When our granddaughter Breanna, comes to visit, she asks for carrot-sticks, raisins, yogurt, vegetables and fruit juices. She doesn't ask for candy or junk food and never asks for soda. She knows none of these exist in our house anyway and has been taught the hazards of bad foods. She now goes around to people's tables in restaurants, informing everyone what effects the foods they are eating, or drinking have on their health. She is five years of age. She has been taught at an early age and has grown to love healthy foods.

Clean out the cupboards. Get rid of the garbage. If its not around, it can't be eaten. You don't just one day say, "You can't have this." Give them a reason, a healthy reason. Teach your children the values of nutrition and eating healthy. I know you are wanting this knowledge because you are reading this book. And if you are this far and hung in for this long, I praise you. You are going to be a healer and knowledge giver. You are going to save lives.

"We have to be the examples for the children."
We grownups must "walk the walk" if we are going to "talk the talk." If we don't, we can't expect our children to. Set an example. Be their hero. These are your children. Take care of them, as Mother Nature takes care of her own.

VEGETARIAN vs. OMNIVOR

I never try to push vegetarianism on anyone. Being a vegetarian isn't <u>for</u> everyone. Vegetarianism was introduced to England in the eighteenth century by Dr. William Lambe. In 1847 the London Vegetarian Society was founded.

There are three basic classifications of vegetarians: "Vegan" that eat nothing made from any animals or products from animals, at all. "Lacto-vegetarians" that drink milk, eat butter and cheese and third, we have the "Lacto-ovo-vegetarian" who are like number two but, whom also eats eggs.

There are many varied reasons why one might choose to become a vegetarian. Some may be for animal rights. Some have been told to eat that way for blood type, while others are doing it on the quest for health. Then, there are those who just want to walk a different path, make a statement or are just doing it because their best friend talked them into it, and they may not have a clue as to why or what they are really doing. But, whatever the reason being in doing so, in my opinion, vegetarianism is the healthier way of eating for humans, for several various reasons.

1. Our digestive enzymes are not strong enough to break down animal protein completely.
2. Our digestive system is three times longer than any carnivore on the planet allowing meat to lay and putrefy, eventually polluting the entire system.
3. Our teeth are not constructed for meat mastication as are true carnivores.

Though being a vegetarian can be quite fun, rewarding and not much to worry about food combining, it does come with some warnings. Inadequate intake of Vitamin B-12 is probably at the top of the list. Our body doesn't synthesis this vitamin and must be acquired through food consumption. Vitamin **B12** is a nutrient that helps keep the body's nerve and blood cells healthy and helps make DNA, the genetic material in all cells. Vitamin **B12** also helps prevent a type of anemia called megaloblastic anemia that makes people tired and weak. **Pernicious anemia** is low iron caused by not enough B-12 reserve to uptake iron. It helps keep bones healthy and helps prevent birth defects. It has many roles and is very crucial to human health. Keep this in mind.

Zinc deficiency is another problem faced by the vegetarian. Not only has the zinc content in our soil greatly diminished, a large consumption of foods rich in phytates (phytic acid), such as beans, rice and legumes, actually bind zinc and other minerals in the digestive tract. Fermentation process neutralizes these phytates. External fermentation. (Not fermentation in your gut from improper food combining.) Another phytate neutralizing technique is sprouting. Include sprouted grains, nuts and seeds in ALL diets.

The most over-publicized problem facing the "vegetarian" is adequate **protein** intake. Let me clear this up for you.

First of all, meat protein is very hard on the human digestive system as we have already discussed, whereas, vegetable protein is very compatible or "user-friendly" with the human organism.

Assuming your digestive tract is completely clear, your pH's are perfect and your digestive enzymes are little cannibalistic, exploding dynamos. On any given day, with the most optimal human functioning systems, the most meat protein you will ever be able to assimilate is 25%. Vegetable protein, on the other hand, is 85% assimilable.

Another lesser problem, but still an important one faced by the vegetarian is: no one vegetable by itself is a **complete protein**, meaning they do not contain the eight essential proteins the body cannot synthesis and must be obtained from outside sources. I'm about to present you with evidence that this information is simply NOT true. There are accumulated data facts from the USDA National Nutrient Database for Standard Refence, that anyone can look up and see for yourself. Eggs are NOT the only source of complete protein.

PROTEIN FACTS

1. We only need 2.5–11% of our daily total calories from protein. By calories, vegetables provide 22% protein, beans 28% and grains 13%. This amount is easily supplied by vegetables.
2. As far as vegetables being an <u>incomplete protein</u>:
   When we compare the USDA food charts of the requirements

of each plant-based food, we find beans are a complete protein. Tomatoes are a complete protein. Carrots are a complete protein. Almost every plant is a complete protein.

3. There is no such thing as food with NO protein. All food has some amount of protein.

The recommended daily allowance (RDA) for protein was thought to be, 65 grams per day for an adult. The new and improved version is more like 15 grams. This is quite a drop, but evidence shows the original figure to be an extreme taxation on the human digestive system and especially the kidneys, if the source is being that of animal.

Naturally, an athlete or body builder will require larger quantities. I feel the protein needs of a normal working adult to be in the 30-gram range. A properly planned out vegetarian diet will easily supply adequate and complete protein requirements.

Another good way to supplement the vegetarian's protein requirements is through a good vegetable protein drink. Capra Goat Whey is one of the finest protein powder for the non-vegan vegetarian.

But, bottom line, vegetarianism is an art. Though it can be very healthy when done correctly, it can be just as detrimental to one's health if done inadequately. Eat a wide variety and colors of vegetables and fruits to obtain the complete spectrum of nutrients. This is the key.

Nearly every vegetarian cookbook you pick up is riddled with cheese this, sugar that, sour cream, whipping cream and stir-fry, stir-fry, stir-fry. This is not eating healthy. This is not vegetarianism. This is simply avoiding eating meat.

First, decide why exactly it is you are becoming a vegetarian. Then, learn the art. Learn food combining and where and how you get all your essential nutrients. Don't just stop eating meat.

Omnivore is just a polite word for scavenger. "Something or someone that eats anything and everything in sight." Let's face it, most humans don't just eat meat. They eat a wide variety of foods and some things that maybe should not even be classified in that category. For now, let's use the polite form and call an "Omnivorous" diet one that includes any and all foods, minus the ones that are totally devoid of nutrients and those ladened with toxins. We'll leave those foods for the "Scavengers."

So, we have chosen to be an Omnivore. That means we will be eating meat and dairy, as well as fruits and vegetables. Let's decide to be a healthy Omnivore. We will choose our meats wisely, buying only organic, antibiotic-free, free range chicken and turkey, anything but farm-raised fish. We will use the preparation methods of baking, broiling or grilling. We will NEVER fry anything, whether it may be organic or not. This will assure we are never putting molecularly-altered, free-radical ladened, saturated fats into our bloodstream. We, as meat eaters, will be consuming complete proteins and a wide spectrum of necessary vitamins and minerals.

Though you won't ever hear me say, "Be a vegetarian," you will hear me say over and over again, "stay away from beef." Not because it doesn't taste good, but because its nearly impossible for the human body to digest. Our enzymes just aren't strong enough to break it down effectively. Unless you periodically cleanse it out, it lays there, in your intestines, with the thirty feet of curves and hair-pin turns, putrefying and polluting your bloodstream, which then visits everywhere else in your body with the same pollution. And like ALL meats, if its commercially raised, its full of antibiotics, steroids and growth hormones. If you were to lay this book down right now and go have you a big ol' juicy steak, unless you give it some help with a cleanse, it will be completely exiting your body in full just about five years from now. That's a fact. Beef is that hard to digest and it takes a long time to remove all the residue from your blood stream and tissues. You will assimilate nutrients from beef but are they worth the risk?

Pork is the other "stay away from the rest of your life meat." The Bible even warns us of the filthiness of the meat of swine. But, it never got around to telling exactly why. Here's the science behind it. Its not because they lay around in the mud all day. Many animals, including your household pets like to do that. Heck, sometimes I might like doing it. The reason is: Pork is the only hoofed animal on the planet with an extra gland placed right in the middle of its front paws so, everything the pig walks through goes straight into its bloodstream, soaks into the tissues and doesn't come out. You can't cook it out.

Here's a fun one for you: Take a porkchop, cooked, raw,

organic or not, doesn't matter. Put it in a pan and pour a can of Coca-Cola over it. Set it outside, because you don't want what is going to take place to do so in your house. Twenty-four hours later, that chop will be covered with maggots and worms. I won't say anymore about it. I'll just let you draw your own conclusions.

I'm just no fun, am I? And never, ever, eat animal entrails. These are the dirtiest parts of the animal. The liver filters all the toxins, poisons, germs and bacteria that's ever gone into the animal. I don't need to tell you <u>what</u> goes through there. The kidneys, another poison filter. This is where the uric acids and all the broken-down poisons the liver just got finished with are sent. The nutritional value of these so thought of, delectable, is not worth the pollutants and poisons you will be introducing into your body. Bowels? Come on! Nature didn't put these filters in animals because the stuff they are filtering out was good for them. I doubt seriously these animals were put through a "full body" detox before butchering.

Not to completely spoil the party, but commercially raised chicken is another one to stay away from. At our health retreat, we enjoy many different people from many different walks of life and sometimes they have a story or two to tell. Some of them can be the most grotesquely disgusting stories you could ever imagine, especially from the refer-haulers. (I'm talking truck drivers that pull refrigerated trailers, for some of you herbalists out there who's eyes started getting all huge and everything!) Our license plate is actually "HERB DR." You think that doesn't turn a few policemen's heads? Our other license plate is "NAT DOC" but that sounds more like I operate on bugs or something. Anyway, I kinda got off the subject.

We have been informed, on numerous occasions, that nearly every chicken that goes down the slaughter-house conveyor belt has a tumor of some sort cut off and thrown in buckets kept under the belt, to go into pet food. This is where we get term "and meat bi-products." Bi-products can and are many times, tumors. The non-health minded pet food companies use the 4D principle. The majority of the products going into the foods are: Diseased, Decomposed, Decayed and Dead, Now, the dead part, I can understand as long as it didn't die from a disease.

Besides all that, commercially raised chickens are pumped full of antibiotics and growth hormones so they will mature in one forth the time Nature intended and they are given cheap feed made from decayed animal parts.

We had another gentleman who hauled beef tell us of a meat-packing plant he pulled up to, and observed a corral out back full of very sickly looking cows, barely able to stand. When he asked what the cows were doing out there, another gentleman told him, "These cows are diseased and were waiting for a truck to come and take them away.

Two hours later, the corral was empty and there hadn't been one single truck go in or out of the plant in the last two hours since our informants arrival, as he had been sitting and watching the front gate the whole time he was there. Where'd they go? Who knows? Who wants to know? We'd better!

The same gentleman was hauling a load of pork at 12 degrees F. The haul was to a city in Texas, where the pork would then be transferred to another truck, to be transported to its final destination six hours into Mexico. Now, the thing to remember here is: if the meat raised up a mere 5 degrees, the shipment would be lost, as the meat would begin thawing itself through heat evaporation.

Now, here comes the transfer truck, also with a big refrigerated trailer. The only thing different about this trailer was the big empty hole where the refrigeration unit was supposed to be. After the meat had been transferred, which took an hour in itself, it was to be another six-hour journey into Mexico in 110-degree weather. Its final destination was the plant of a very well- known "Pork and Beans" company. (FDA approved)

Let's get back to the chicken. We have some more clients who are organic farmers and formerly being cattle and poultry farmers. They were asked to tour a chicken-processing plant and in doing so, noticed a very strange odor coming from a huge vat in the center of the room. As they approached the vat, they were informed, "None of the chickens are able to be processed fast enough and most begin to rot and turn blue. We found that, by soaking them in a vat of chlorine, we're able to bleach then back white again." "

Same folks again, had toured a beef-processing plant and witnessed a cow so weak from illness, it was unable to pick itself off the floor. Now, it's a Federal Law that one cannot slaughter, process and sell a cow that is not standing. So, what did they do? They drove in this little tiny fork-lift. That was barely able to squeeze down the aisle, slid the forks on either side of the diseased cow, raised her to a standing position and slaughtered her. There have recently been several television shows aired on this subject. But, this was from a personal eye-witness account. I might add one thing, this particular person of whom I speak, was head of animal research at a very prestigious university.

Chickens are programmed to lay one egg when the sun comes up. Now, to fool Mother Nature and trick the chickens into laying two eggs daily instead of one, the chickens are kept in a dark room, the lights are turned on, then off, then on again. The chickens think its morning and lay two eggs in one day. Problem is, the eggshells are so thin and fragile, they have to be processed with chemicals to make them strong enough to be handled. Sodium silicate is one such product.

Turkeys, to make their breasts wider and appear fuller, are kept in a cage so short, they are unable to completely stand up for the duration of their whole life.

All this is regulated and approved by our Food and Drug Administration.

Did you know: Monsanto has blue ears of corn that are nearly two feet long? If that's not genetic modification…

With chicken wings being such a popular item, the same University I mentioned earlier, is raising chickens with four and six wings. True story. They also raise, what my patient referred to as "Dolly Parton" chickens, their breast being so large, they can't hold themselves up to eat. What are these people doing? Guys, I thought you were supposed to be looking out for our health? Vegetarianism is looking better all the time, huh?

Here's the point I want to make here. If you are going to eat chicken and turkey, by free-range, grain-fed, "Certified Organic" chicken and turkey. It can be purchased in most grocery stores. If possible, I would go one step further and buy local. Get to know the supplier. That way you know what you are getting. If you're "DEAD" set on eating animal, its well worth the extra trouble of finding a good source. Its worth your life.

PLANT-BASED vs. MEAT-BASED DIET COMPARISON

The Cold Hard Facts

I will present this factual information and you can do with it as you like. I said I will never tell a person to go vegetarian, but…

As I stated earlier, the myth about meat and eggs being the only source of complete protein, is a lie. ALL protein originates from plants. The animals, get their protein from the plants they eat. The pigs, cows and chickens are simply the go-between that passes the protein from one source to another.

That being said, let's get into some pertinent facts.

1. Vegetarians acquire 70 percent more protein than they actually need.
2. Every plant is a complete protein.
3. The strongest man in the world, Patrik Baboumian, is a total vegan. He's said to be strong as an ox. Ever see an ox eat meat? The gorilla, the elephant, the rhino; are ALL strictly vegetarian. They have more strength and protein mass than any human being on the planet, all from a plant-based diet.

Blood Flow Restriction

The "endothelial lining" of the arterial walls regulate blood flow throughout the body. It knows when to dilate if a particular organ or muscle is in need of more blood supply, as in the example of exercise. If impaired, blood flow can't increase.

1. One hamburger lowers the endothelial function by 27 percent.
2. Plants increase endothelial function and blood flow.
3. It has been proven, drinking beet juice before an event increased the cyclist's stamina and ability by 27 percent and the weight-lifter's max limit increased by 19 percent.

Inflammation

1. Meat contains inflammatory molecules such as New 5-6C, Endotoxins and Feme iron.
2. One milligram of Feme iron a day raises the risk of Coronary Heart Disease by 27 percent.

3. One hamburger patty contains 2 mg of Feme iron.
4. Same portion of tuna contains 1.5 mg and chicken 1.3 mg.
5. One hamburger increases inflammation by 70 percent.
6. Animal-based products increase soreness in muscles and joints, creating inflammation which impairs and delays recovery.
7. A plant-based diet can reduce inflammation by 29 percent in 3 weeks.
8. Meat changes the healthy gut bacteria while stimulating inflammation-causing bacteria to propagate inflammatory mediators such as TMAO (Trimethylamine-N-Oxide) and C-Reactive Protein (indicates the possibility of a serious illness being present).
9. Science has proven that ALL meat, whether grass-fed, organic and drug-free or not, causes inflammation and aging.

Heart Disease +

1. Animal products cause plaque to form in the coronary arteries. This, in turn, impairs blood flow resulting in impeding the heart's ability to keep up with the demands of the body.
2. The actual animal protein (not just the iron), which includes eggs, milk, cheese and meat, institute and immediate process at the chemical level. The preserving, cooking or digesting of animal products create bi-products called "amines." These are highly corrosive to the cardiovascular system.
3. Plant based diets reduce the risk
4. A high meat-based diet raises the risk by 75% of premature death from ALL causes.
5. Meat-based diet raises the risk of death by cancer 400-500% in the form of colon, prostate and breast cancer, as well as type II diabetes.
6. Vegetarians, eating one plate of chicken a week, triples their risk of colon cancer. (Why would they do that? For test results.)
7. Amino acids from animal products make red blood cells rev up and multiply at a much faster rate, resulting in a 40% risk increase of prostate cancer.

For Men Only; Maybe Not

Here are some facts in regards to our little buddy that swings freely between the uprights: our dude-piston, Johnson, heat-sinking moisture missile, ding-dong McDork or whatever euphemism you use to refer to yours.

As we all know, blood engorgement is what raises our proud flagpole to the "at-attention" state. The more blood flow, the harder it gets. During sleep, men have repeated involuntary erections throughout the entire night. With that information in mind…

1. Two hours after eating meat, your blood becomes opaque or cloudy with animal fat and remains in this state for 6-7 hours.
2. A plant-based diet produces consistently clear blood- no fat.
3. Compared to the results of just one day of meat-based meals, the one day of plant-based diet increased the circumference of the erection between 9% and 13% and the frequency of nightly between 303% and 500%. This is due to the restriction of blood flow from meat, compared to the non-restriction of blood-flow from a plant-based diet.

"Real Men Eat Meat"

Is nothing more than marketing propaganda based on selling technique, not reality. There are companies hired to produce studies that deny the truth of the original studies. These studies are designed to provide propaganda for new and confusing ad campaigns from cigarettes to foods to medicines. It all ends up in the hands of Big Pharma anyway, to treat the conditions caused by the misinformation which led to the disease you now have as a result of the mis-information put out by the media, owned by Big Pharma companies to begin with.

For Women and Men, as Well

" Hormones and Meat and Weight Loss"

1. Soy, that once touted "hormone wrecker" actually contains Phyto-estrogens that have proven to control estrogen levels rather than disrupt them.
2. Animal meat, especially red meat, contains real estrogen that

can actually throw estrogen hormones completely out-of-balance.

3. One glass of cow's milk can increase men's estrogen levels by 26% in 1 hour, while dropping the testosterone by 18%.
4. Cortisol, the stress hormone we talked about under adrenal repair, rears its ugly head once again. It is linked to decreased muscle-mass and increased body fat.
5. Going a plant-based diet from a meat-based diet reduces one's cortisol levels by a 27% average.
6. While during an 8-week weight-training trial, the normal carb intake persons gained 2.9 lbs. more muscle mass while the low carb persons lost muscle.

The Differences in Carnivorous and Vegetarian Species

1. Carnivore teeth are scissor-shaped for ripping meat from bones while vegetarians teeth are square and flat for grinding, as in human beings.
2. The carnivore intestinal tract is 2 times the length of the body for quick evacuation of the meat to avoid rotting and putrefying. On the other hand, the vegetarian intestinal tract is 6 times the length of the body, resulting in longer digesting time for extracting more nutrients from the plant food.
3. Vegetarian enzymes are not nearly strong enough to break down animal proteins. Humans have such enzymes. Our bodies were designed to rely on the intact plant enzymes digesting themselves, saving us the expenditure of energy otherwise depleted from the manufacturing of digestive enzymes.
4. The energy loss from a meat-based diet compared to plant-based energy gain, can be explained like this: When eating a plant-based diet with 85% of the enzymes still intact, one creates energy from the explosiveness of the digestive enzymes colliding with the plant enzymes. Secondly, this, in turn, absconds one's self from the exhausting task of having to manufacture the horrendous amount of enzymes needed to digest the meat. So you see, the vegetarian is gaining energy two-fold, while the carnivore is losing energy.

Various Fad Diets

Regardless of the verification or opinions from the creators of the many various "fad diets," Harvard University and The Max Planck Institute, using breakthroughs in technology, have been able to verify that our ancestors were nearly "total" vegetarians.

I'm not going to go dissect these diets. You can do that for yourself. There are definite health benefits from the Keto Diet and the Paleo Diet, and you will lose weight while adjusting your glucose. But the facts are:
1. You need carbs for fuel. Our brains use nothing but glucose for fuel.
2. Animal protein causes all the previously mentioned physiological side-effects from heart disease diabetes, hormone imbalances and cancer.
3. Animal products are acidic as well as mucous-forming.
4 Humans can't utilize the majority of the protein contained within the meat.
5. The detriments to a meat-based diet far out weight the few benefits obtained from animal products.

Factual Effects of Raising Cattle for Food
1. Three quarters of ALL the agricultural land in the world is used for livestock production.
2. The biggest source of habitat destruction is associated with livestock production.
3. Dairy, eggs, meat and fish hatcheries use 83% of the world's farmlands and yet, provide only 18% of the world's calories.
4. Livestock requires so much land because they consume 6 times more protein than they produce.
5. Plant foods to feed the 70 billion animals consumed per year creates the leading drivers of deforestation.
6. Twenty-five percent of the rivers never reach the ocean due to so much water being removed to produce animal feed.
7. It takes 2400 liters of embedded water to produce one hamburger, due to crop-growing for feed for these animals.
8. Twenty-seven percent of ALL fresh water supplies go to produce animal foods.
9. Because water consumption, there is the problem of water pollution. Farm animals in the U.S. alone, produce 50 times

more waste than the entire human population.
10. Livestock is responsible for 15% of all the man-
    made emissions, globally. In perspective, that's the same as
    all the forms of transportation in the world. This includes:
    planes, cars, trucks, trains, ships and motorcycles.
11. U.S. meat consumption is three times the world average.
12. Shifting gears from a meat-based diet to a plant-based diet
    would reduce emissions by 73%.
13. A plant- based diet would save approximately 1 million liters
    of water per person; per year.
14. This would also free up a total land-mass area the size of
    Africa.

Human Organs and Systems that need Carbohydrates
1. Without proper glucose levels, your entire nervous system can
   develop central nervous system disease.
2. Your brain thrives on glucose as its main source of fuel.
3. All your 650 muscles need glucose to operate.
4. Glucose is needed in cellular respiration to produce ATP
5. Animal meat has a very low source of glucose.

The last alert I would like to address with any chosen method of eating: The soil bacteria that actually creates vitamin B-12 is being destroyed with chemicals and poisons and must be additionally supplemented by both the vegetarian and carnivore.

There you have it. Take what you like, leave what you don't. Each of us have our own reasons and I am not going to attempt to convince anyone of anything. It's your choice.

I personally go with the vegan route. I am planning on living at least 150 years and I will do it!

I shall leave this subject with one final thought: Humans and animals synthesis proteins using the 20 amino acids available and both can make eleven of these twenty amino acids. But there are nine amino acids known as "essential" amino acids that humans and animals cannot make. These must be obtained from an external source. So where do the essential amino acids come from in the first place? They come from plants. Plants can manufacture ALL the amino acids, including the essential amino acids. In my opinion, that makes <u>plants</u> the King of proteins.

CHAPTER 7
DEATH BY INGESTION

FDA APPROVED, DOESN'T MEAN IT'S SAFE

One third of what we eat keeps us alive, the other two thirds, keep the doctor alive. Man creates either health or disease at the table. We eat foods that have been overcooked, over-processed beyond the point of any nutritional value, genetically altered and loaded with chemicals, preservatives, food coloring, hydrogenated oils and DEATH.

The FDA has okayed many foods, additives and drugs throughout the years that have later (some known at the time of approval) been proven detrimental or deadly for human consumption. Unfortunately, we usually find out this information much too late, after many persons have become ill or have died.

We all know commercial meats are saturated with drugs of all kinds to make the animals grow faster, bigger and make it through contagious diseases until they can be processed and sold at the market. The FDA knows these drugs to be extremely detrimental to everyone's health, including death. Still, they are being okayed by the FDA.

We know, they know, alcohol causes brain damage, liver damage, kills thousands of people each year, directly and indirectly, and it has the FDA's blessing. Cigarettes, another fine example; lung cancer, emphysema, heart disease, all are proven killers, still approved! Many food additives are proven carcinogens, detrimental to human health, but they're still pumped into our food and completely approved by our friends and health guardians, the FDA.

Aspartame-"M.S. symptoms, neurological disorders.

Aspirin- Leaky gut syndrome, the cause of most M.S. and
      Lupus.

Hydrogenated oils-clogged arteries

Corn Syrup- addictive fattening agent, causes diabetes

I'll get into all of this later. But so many of our foods are completely devoid of anything useful to our health. Some are absolute poisons and yet, we continue to consume them without a care in the world, not a second thought about it. Why? Because deep in the back of our minds, we have the FDA's promise that these foods are safe to eat and good for us, as well. And even deeper in the backs of our minds, we don't want to believe any differently, "cause we like this food"!

Drink milk for healthy bones. Eat cheese to lose weight. The milk is pasteurized, dead of most nutrients. The cheese is wreathing with mold, fungus and saturated trans-fats. Take this pill to get well, then this one to combat the ten new side effects that come along with the first one. Suck on a cigarette to be cool. That will go real stylish, especially with that new iron lung you'll be hossin' around just to breathe. Emphysema and lung cancer are really cool too. Just ask the people dying from it. Drip greasy hamburger down the front of your shirt and look all macho while you're punchin' the head of your hula-doll on your dashboard. And don't forget to wash it all down with a big ol' glass of refreshing, enamel-eating, battery-cleaning, soda pop. Mmmmm, and its all good for you, as it should be. Its all been FDA approved.

I have what? I'm supposed to weigh how much? I have how long to live? What do you mean, my heart is about to explode? You need to take out my what?

Keep eating and taking all these FDA approved products and these are the questions you'll be dealing with.

Latest governmental statistics are: 699,997 deaths from heart dis-ease, 553,251 from cancer and 975,000 from pharmaceutical drug-related causes. Most of these deaths, caused by these FDA approved products could and absolutely should have been avoided.

Did you know: 370,000 person die each year by "iatrogenesis" or medical mistakes. And do they go to jail? No, they get paid. Do the folks at Monsanto, making carcinogenic products that have killed persons and still they continually produce them, go to jail? No. Do any of these people get tried for murder? Isn't that what they are doing? Is this not a form of pre-meditated murder? These facts aren't my opinions, they are proven statistics.

To sum it up, eat sensibly, eat healthy, so much that your doctor couldn't possibly find anything to give you a drug for and you'll avoid being one of those statistics.

CHEMICALS IN OUR FOODS

Let's talk about names and side effects of some of the more common, everyday chemicals of preservatives you might see on cans and labels, and find in your foods, even though they aren't listed on the labels. Not ALL ingredients are required by law to be listed. A lot has to do with loop holes, word trickery and the bending of the rules. Many chemicals (all, of course, being man-made) and many from petroleum, are simply the by-products of a contract to produce some chemical or petroleum company some extra change.

Artificial Flavorings- comprising one of the largest and most important categories of food additives. Artificial flavorings mask the absence of more "natural" flavorings and ALL being concocted of synthetic, man-made chemicals. For this reason alone, one should not ingest anything labeled "Artificially Flavored." Tests or no tests, you should know by now, you don't mix organic matter and chemicals together and expect anything but BAD to happen. All chemicals are a detriment to the organic body. By the way, many have been tested and many have been shown to cause birth defects, liver damage, brain damage and allergic reactions such as migraines, irritable bowel syndrome, cancer and mutations.

Amyl-Alcohol- It is used to imitate brandy flavoring in numerous commercial bakery goods. Medical tests have proven that 30 cc can cause death. Smaller doses can cause kidney damage. This is one of the ingredients that fall under the "artificial flavorings" category. By law, it does not have to be specified on the label. This chemical is also used as a varnish solvent.

Allyl Isothiocyanate- Adds artificial mustard flavor to sauces. It was used in the making if poisonous gases in World War I. It has been shown to produce slow healing ulcers and death.

Butyric Acid- Also used to impart a butter flavor to baked goods. Used in industry to de-calcify hides and is an ingredient in varnishes.

Ethyl Formate- This gives baked goods a rum flavor and is also used as a tobacco fungicide as well as a solvent for nitrocellulose.

It gets even better. I want to start with some of the stuff that goes into one of our favorite treats. Kids want it, grownups want it. You scream, I scream, we all scream for…you got it, ICE CREAM! That wonderful, delectable, mouth-watering, cool you down on a hot summer's day, frozen fantasy of flavor. Well, let's just look at some of the chemicals that go into this tantalizing A-LA-MODE. Now remember, these are all "FDA approved."

Diethyl glycol- a cheap chemical used as an emulsifier in eggs. Many fatal poisonings have been linked to DG.

Piperonal- extensively used as a substitute for vanilla. Also used to KILL LICE!

Aldehyde C17- "sounds like germ warfare," is used to flavor cherry ice cream. This liquid is used in aniline dyes, plastics and rubber. Nothing like a little rubber-blubber.

Ethyl acetate- used to achieve pineapple flavor. Also serves as a cleaner for leather and textiles and as a solvent for lacquer.

Butyraldehyde- gives you that various "nutty-like" flavor and is commonly an ingredient in rubber cement.

Amyl acetate- gives your ice-cram that banana flavor and is used commercially as an oil paint solvent.

Benzyl acetate- gives us strawberry flavor, also used as a solvent for plastics.

We probably all have a whole storage shed full of chemicals and ice-cream additives sitting there, just waiting to be concocted, frozen and A-LA-MODED and didn't even know it!
Mind you, not ALL brands of ice cream use this garbage,

mainly the cheaper ones. But don't be caught off guard simply because you paid more for the product. Just because it costs more, doesn't mean you get more. Be careful what you put into that thing! It might be smilin' at one end but might end up frownin' at the other. Freeze a smoothie. Its healthy and good.

THE COLORS OF OUR FOOD

FD&C- By law, these letters have to be put on a label. But, by law, they DO NOT have to tell us what these letters stand for. FD&C are food colorings the FDA has "Certified." Consequently. The FD&C certified colorings are the ones we have to be worried about. Imagine that! Uncertified colors aren't considered to be AS dangerous. But the certified colors are man-made chemicals and are universally accepted as "CARCINOGENS." So, the FDA is merely "certifying" that these products CAUSE CANCER. Why are they still putting them in our food? Food and Drug "Certified" carcinogens! Its almost as if they're seeing how stupid we are and just how much they can get away with, by putting right under our noses. FD&C means, "Its in here. You are eating this at your own risk, not ours. We warned you." But they don't say what they are warning you of.

The United States is basically the ONLY country in the world that allows the use of food coloring agents in their food. Again, just because the FDA approves something doesn't mean its safe to eat.

Remember, many items are products of "payola." Here's one example: **Red #4** was about to be banned entirely from food, due to the fact it was proven to harm the adrenal glands and bladder. But, the maraschino cherry lobbyists convinced (paid) the FDA that one only eats a few maraschino cherries at a time and would not ingest enough Red #4 to cause harm. Now, I know most of us as kids, if given half a chance, would eat a whole freakin' half gallon of maraschino cherries. Are these people's brains truly in their pockets? And what well known body part do the pockets border? Ahhh, that explains it!

Yellow #6- used to color butter, can cause blindness. **Red #2**- used to impart a striking cherry red to certain soft drinks, candies, ice cream, cherries (cherries?) baked goods and even sausage. No…not sausage!...was banned from the Soviet Union on the grounds it induced cancer.

Now, mind you, these have ALL been FDA "Certified" as healthy to ingest.

"Just because the FDA says its healthy, doesn't make it safe to eat."

Here's the red flag to be very aware of: When you see FD&C on a label, you are being warned this product contains colors that absolutely, having been laboratory tested and proven, beyond a shadow of a doubt, to cause cancer.

Note: These FD&C's have supposedly been recently banned by the FDA. But, read carefully. They're still in there in products produced under the wire!

MORE CHEMICALS AND PRESERVATIVES

Aspartame- Artificial sweetener.

I was going to put this in my own words, but I do not think I could state it anymore convincing than the email I received on May 09, 2007, on this dreadfully dangerous chemical, many persons such as diabetics, have been led to believe was a healthy choice. Many of you have also already read this same article. But for those who have not seen or heard this information, I would now like to share it with you. Here it is, in full.

SWEET POISON

SWEET, BUT POISON- A MUST READ- Diabetics don't despair. Read thru to the end.

In October of 2001, my sister started having a hard time getting around. Walking was a major chore. It took everything she had to get out of bed; she was in so much pain.

By March 2002, she had undergone several tissue and muscle biopsies and was on 24 prescription medications. The doctors could not determine what was wrong with her. She was in so much pain, and so sick, she just knew she was dying. She put her house, bank accounts, life insurance, etc., in her oldest daughter's name and made sure that her younger children were to be taken care of. She also wanted her last hooray, so she planned a trip to Florida (basically in a wheelchair) for March 22nd.

On March 19, I called to ask how her most recent tests went, and she said they didn't believe she had M.S. I recalled an article a friend of mine e-mailed to me and I asked my sister if she drank diet soda? She told me that she did. As a matter of fact, she was getting ready to crack one open that moment. I told her not to open it and to stop drinking the diet soda. I e-mailed her the article my friend, a lawyer, had sent. My sister called me within 32 hours after our phone conversation and told me she had stopped drinking the diet soda AND she could walk! The muscle spasms went away. She didn't feel 100% but she sure felt a lot better. She told me she was going to her doctor with the article and would call me when she got home.

Well, she called me and said her doctor was amazed! He is going to call all of his MS patients to find out if they consumed artificial sweeteners of any kind.

In a nutshell, she was going to be poisoned by the Aspartame in the diet soda and literally dying a slow and painful death. When she got to Florida, March 22, all se had to take was one pill and that was the pill for the Aspartame poisoning.

If it says "SUGAR FREE" on the label,
DON'T EVEN THINK ABOUT IT!

Here's the article that saved her life:

I have spent several days lecturing at the WORLD ENVIRONMENTAL CONFERENCE on" Aspartame," marketed as "Nutra-sweet," "Equal" and "Spoonful." In the keynote address by the EPA, it was announced that in the United States in 2001, there is an epidemic of Multiple Sclerosis and Systemic Lupus. It was difficult to determine exactly what toxin was causing this to be rampant. I stood up and said I was there to lecture on exactly that subject.

I will explain why Aspartame is so dangerous: When the

temperature of this sweetener exceeds 86 degrees F, the wood alcohol in Aspartame converts to formaldehyde and then to formic acid, which in turn, causes metabolic acidosis. Formic acid is the poison found in the sting of fire ants. The methanol toxicity mimics, among other conditions, multiple sclerosis and systemic lupus .Many people were being diagnosed in error. Although multiple sclerosis is not a death sentence, methanol toxicity is! Systemic Lupus has become almost as rampant as Multiple Sclerosis, especially with Diet Coke and Pepsi drinkers.

The victims usually does not know the Aspartame is the culprit. He or she continues its use, irritating the Lupus to such a degree that it may become a life-threatening condition. We have seen patients with Systemic Lupus became asymptomatic once taken off diet sodas.

In cases of those diagnosed with Multiple Sclerosis, most of the symptoms disappear. We've seen many cases where vision loss returned, and hearing loss improved markedly. This also applies to cases of tinnitus and fibromyalgia.

During a lecture, I said, "If you are using Aspartame (NutraSweet, Equal, Spoonful, etc.) and you suffer from fibromyalgia symptoms, spasms, shooting pains, numbness in your legs, cramps, vertigo, dizziness, headaches, Tinnitus, joint pain, unexplainable depression, anxiety attacks, slurred speech, blurred vision or memory loss, you probably have Aspartame poisoning! People were jumping up during the lecture saying, "I have some of these symptoms. Is it reversable?" Yes! Yes! Yes! Stop drinking diet sodas and be alert for Aspartame on food labels. Many products are fortified with it. This is a serious problem.

Dr. Espart (one of my speakers) remarked that so many people seem to be symptomatic for MS and during one of his visits to hospice, a nurse stated that six of her friends, who were heavy Diet Coke addicts, had all been diagnosed with MS. This is beyond coincidence! Diet soda in NOT a diet product. It is chemically altered, multiple SODIUM (salt) and ASPARTAME containing product that actually makes you crave carbohydrates. It is far more likely to make you GAIN weight!

These products also contain formaldehyde, which stores in the fat cells, particularly in the hips and thighs. Formaldehyde is an absolute toxin and is used primarily to preserve tissue specimens. Many products we use every day contain this chemical, but we SHOULD NOT store it in our body!

Dr. H.J Roberts stated in his lectures that once free of the "diet products" and with no significant increase in exercise; his patients lost an average of 19 pounds over a trial period.

Aspartame is especially dangerous for diabetics. We found that some physicians, who believe that they had a patient with retinopathy, in fact, had symptoms caused by Aspartame. The Aspartame drives the blood sugar out of control. Thus, diabetic may suffer acute memory loss due to the fact that aspartic acid and phenylalanine are neurotoxic when taken without the other amino acids necessary for a good balance.

Treating diabetes is all about balance. Especially with diabetics, the Aspartame passes the blood/brain barrier and it then deteriorates the neurons of the brain, causing various levels of brain damage, seizures, depression, manic depression, panic attacks, uncontrollable anger and rage.

Consumption of Aspartame causes these same symptoms in non-diabetics as well. Diagnosis and observation also reveals that thousands of children diagnosed with ADD and ADHD have had complete turnarounds in their behavior when these chemicals have been removed from their diet. So called "behavioral modification prescription drugs" (Ritalin and others) are no longer needed. Truth be told, they were never needed on the first place! Most of these children were being poisoned on a daily basis with the very foods that were "better for them than sugar."

It is also suspected that the Aspartame in thousands of pallets of Diet Coke consumed by men and women fighting in the Gulf War, may be partially to blame for the well-known Gulf War Syndrome.

Dr. Roberts warns that it can cause birth defects, i.e. intellectual disabilities (mentalretardation in medical terminology) if taken at the time of conception and during early pregnancy. Children are especially at risk for neurological disorders and should NEVER be given artificial sweeteners.

There are many different case histories to relate children suffering grand-mal seizures and other neurological disturbances due to the use of NutraSweet. Unfortunately, it is not always easy to convince people that Aspartame is to blame for their child's illness.

Stevia, which is a sweet herb, NOT A MANUFACTURED ADDITIVE, helps in the metabolism of sugar, which would be ideal for diabetics. It has now been approved by the FDA, but it is well known that for many years, the FDA outlawed this true sweet food, "due to the loyalty of the MONSANTO Chemical Company."

Books on this subject are available: Excitotoxins: The Taste That Kills, by Dr. Russell Blaylock (Health Press 1-800-643-26650 AND: Defense Against Alzheimer's Disease-written by Dr. H.J Roberts, also a diabetic specialist. These two doctors will soon be posting a position paper on the internet with case histories on the deadly effects of Aspartame, according to the American College of Physicians.

"We are talking about a plague of neurological diseases directly caused by the use of this deadly poison.

Herein lies the problem: There were Congressional Hearings when Aspartame was included in 100 different products, and strong objection was made concerning its use. Since this initial hearing, there have been two subsequent hearings, and nothing has been done.

The drug and chemical lobbies have very deep pockets. Sadly, MONSANTO's patent on Aspartame has EXPIRED! There are now, over 5,000 products on the market that contain this deadly chemical and there will be thousands more introduced. Everyone wants a "piece of the Aspartame pie."

I assure you that MONSANTO. The creator of Aspartame, knows how deadly it is. And isn't it ironic that MONSANTO funds, among others, the American Diabetes Association, the American Dietetic Association and the Conference of the American College of Physicians? This has been recently exposed in the New York Times.

These (organizations) cannot criticize and additives or convey their links to MONSANTO because they take away from the food industry and are required to endorse their products.

Senator Howard Metzenbaum wrote and presented a bill that would require label warnings on products containing Aspartame, especially regarding pregnant women, children and infants. The bill would also institute independent studies on the known dangers and the problems existing in the general population regarding seizures, changes in brain chemistry, neurological changes and behavioral symptoms. The bill was killed.

It is known that th powerful drug and chemical lobbies are responsible for this, letting loose the hounds of disease and death on an unsuspecting and uninformed public.

Well, you're informed, now!

YOU HAVE A RIGHT TO KNOW!

(End of e-mail)

If you have anyone with any of these type symptoms, share this info. You may just save their life. Now, let's continue on with more of our FDA approved additives:

Benzoic Acid- This is a preservative in many foods including: drinks, low-sugar products, meat products and cereals. Can temporarily inhibit the function of digestive enzymes. May deplete glycine levels. Avoid if you suffer from asthma, rhinitis, urticaria or other allergies.

BHA (butylated hydroxy anisole)- an unnecessary antioxidant used to combat rancidity in fatty foods. (Not to be confused with the good anti-oxidants, good for one's health) Some examples containing BHA as well as BHT are: breakfast cereals, vegetable oils, shortening, potato chips, chewing gum and many oil-containing products. Both BHA and BHT are proven carcinogens and are known to cause changes in the DNA of cells and one or both are in most prepared food products.

BHT (butylated hydroxytoluene)- also an unnecessary anti-oxidant. Side effects are listed in previous description.

Blue Lake- Carcinogenic, but pretty! (See below section on food colorings)

BVO- Here is one you probably have never heard of and will never see on a label. This chemical keeps oil flavoring in soft drinks from floating to the top. It has been banned in Sweden.

But, Americans keep putting it in their snacks and soft drinks. Totally devoid of nutritional value. This product accumulates in the fatty tissue and has tested out to be a possible carcinogen. ("possibly" means, you can bet on it!)

Caffeine- Everybody's friend and pick-me-up. Though it being a naturally occurring substance of nature, it is added to other products and abused with its affect on the human adrenal system. Coffee, for instance, our own personal cup of energy.
Did you know: with every cup of coffee you consume, you go into deeper "adrenal failure?"

You believe you are consuming energy, when in essence, you are forcing adrenaline to be unnecessarily produced and released into your body. This hormone is reserved for important, life-threatening occasions when you really might need to have adrenaline pumping through your veins, let's say, in the event that someone might be actually trying to HURT YOU! Aside from that, here are some more effects brought on by caffeine consumption:

1. Capillary constriction to the brain, reducing cerebral flow by as much as 30%, meaning blood flow and oxygen to the brain is reduced.
2. Less blood to the brain means less ability to think clearly, less memory retention, as well as oxygen starvation to brain cells, meaning brain cell deterioration. Dementia and Alzheimer's.
3. Causes elevation in heart rate and elevated spikes in hormones.
4. Promotes stomach acidity and increasing the symptoms of peptic ulcers.
5. Promotes nervousness and insomnia.
   In women, the damaging effects are far more numerous, including :
1. Weakening of the bones (caused by over-acidification)
2. Fracture risk
3. Heart disease
4. Anxiety and panic attacks
5. Anemia
6. PMS
7. Menopausal complications

8. Fibromyalgia
9. Chronic fatigue
10. Depression
11. Conception and fertility disorders (men too)
12. Complications during pregnancy and childbirth.

Caffeine has also been shown to cause birth defects such as cleft palates, missing fingers and toes, as well as skull mal-formations.

Calcium Stearate- See under "Stearates" below.

Diethylene Glycol- this has been used to induce cancer in test animals. Manufacturers are well aware of this, but they continue to use it anyway. It is used as additives in breads, rolls, ice cream, shredded coconut, marshmallows, chocolates and jelly-like candies.

Emulsifiers- make water mix with fats in a product and used to replace the product's natural emulsifiers, which have been unnaturally removed via processing. Excess emulsifiers in the body pose a serious threat by disturbing the bio-chemical action of the stomach and intestinal linings. This, in turn, enables ingested poisons to pass more easily into our systems. Emulsifiers increase the intake of iron from foods, concentrating in excess, in the spleen, promoting cirrhosis and cancer of the liver.
    Some emulsifiers cause extreme absorption of vitamin A, which is toxic at high levels and others may increase the uptake of other carcinogenic additives.

Enriched with- This is a good one. This phrase right-off-the-bat is the main clue to stay away from this stuff. It has been enriched, and they are even bragging about it…or so they want you to believe. What they are really doing is hiding the fact that it needed to be enriched, because it has been stripped of all its "natural occurring" nutrients, which must now be replaced or "enriched" as they like to refer. This is a very misleading trick of the words and the mind. Unfortunately, these enriched vitamins are again, synthetic, man-made chemicals that are absolutely and completely UNUSABLE by the human organic organism.

"Fortified" is the other interchangeable brainwashing terminology of worthless, braggadocios BULL! If its "Fortified" or "Enriched" it ain't natural and it ain't healthy! Why did it need fortified? If used in its naturally occurring state, it would still be full of its original nutritional elements. Where'd they go?

Fluoride- Pretty much covered this one earlier. Neurotoxin and by-product from aluminum manufacturer runoff. Causes neurological damage, rots teeth and bones, calcifies pineal gland and is an all-round poison that should NEVER, EVER be consumed.

Hydrogenated and partially hydrogenated oils- are oils that have been subjected to high heat, extreme pressure and exposed to a metal catalyst for a several hour period. The final outcome is a hydrogenated, saturated fat that extends the product's shelf-life without the use of refrigeration. The process of hydrogenation changes the molecular structure of the oils, into an instant barrage of toxins and "free-radicals," totally unusable by the human system. Cotton, being heavily pesticided in the fields, lends Cotton Seed Oil to contain the highest pesticide residue of all the commercial oils. When you see "partially hydrogenated oils" it means it is halfway to the state of clogging your arteries and plasticizing your cell membranes. Stay AWAY from ALL hydrogenated ANYTHINGS!

Magnesium Stearate- See under "stearates" below.

MSG (Monosodium Glutamate)- responsible for what has been called "The Chines Restaurant Syndrome." Shortly after ingesting MSG in Chinese food, MSG intolerant persons would complain of a burning sensation in the back of the neck, migraine headaches and tightness to the chest. It is estimated that some eighty percent of persons in the U.S. have some adverseness or allergies toward MSG. It's the salt seasoning used in many Chinese restaurants and dishes.

HIDDEN SOURCES OF MSG

As discussed previously, the glutamate (MSG) manufacturers and the processed food industries are always on the quest to disguise the MSG added to food. Below is a partial list of the most common names for disguised MSG. Remember also, the powerful excitotoxins, aspartate and L-Cysteine, are frequently added to foods, and according to FDA rules, require NO LABELING AT ALL.

*** Food Additives that ALWAYS contain MSG***
Monosodium Glutamate
Hydrolyzed Vegetable Protein
Hydrolyzed Protein
Hydrolyzed Plant Protein
Plant Protein Extract
Sodium Caseinate
Yeast Extract
Texturized Protein (including TVP)
Hydrolyzed Oat Flour
Autolyzed Yeast
Corn Oil

*** Food Additives that FREQUENTLY Contain MSG***
(these are key words to look for in the ingredients)
Malt Extract
Malt Flavoring
Bouillon
Broth
Stock
Flavoring
Natural Flavors/Flavoring
Natural Beef or Chicken Flavoring
Seasonings
Spices

Food Additives that MAY Contain MSG or Excitotoxins
Carrageenan
Enzymes

Soy Protein Concentrate
Soy Protein Isolate
Whey Protein Concentrate

Olestra (Olean)- A fat-free additive found in fat-free potato chips, fries, corn chips and many other items touting fat-free. It is banned in most countries. It causes gas, bloating, abdominal cramps and anal leakage. It causes malabsorption of fat-soluble vitamins and therefor, by FDA regulations, requires ALL foods containing Olestra (Olean) to be fortified (there it is again) with vitamins, A, D, E and K. But, they still let it slide right on through.

Potassium Bromate- can irritate the lungs. Repeated exposure may cause bronchitis to develop with cough, phlegm, and/or shortness of breath. Repeated exposure to Potassium Bromate may affect the nervous system causing headache, irritability, impaired thinking and personality changes

Used in the U.S. as an oxidizing agent and flour improver. Acts to strengthen the dough and allows it to rise higher.

Potassium Sorbate- See below under Sodium Benzoate.

WHAT ARE WE TRYING TO PRESERVE, ANYWAY?

Sodium Benzoate- and **Potassium Sorbate** are used as a preservative in most of the liquid vitamins sold in health food stores or Multi-Level Marketing distributors. What's the sole function of a preservative? It kills everything alive in the product so it can sit for weeks or months on a store or warehouse shelf without spoiling. If it kills everything alive in the product, what do you think it's doing inside your body? Manufactured in the use of: margarine, jellies, carbonated drinks, candy, fruit juices, jams, pickles, mincemeat and many, many other items.

Dr. Harvey Wiley M'D. "Father of the Pure Food and Drug Act" of 1906, later to become the organization now known as the FDA, tried to get President Coolidge to ban the use of sodium benzoate in food items. It should have been banned as a preservative at that time, but food adulterators radically protested to the Secretary of Agriculture, allowing for the continued poisonous usage of this extremely harmful preservative today. It now graces the FDA's "GRAS" list, Generally Recognized as Safe, along with hundreds of other chemicals that shouldn't be allowed in our foods and supplements.

Since the whole purpose of adding a preservative to a food is to make it unfit for insects and mold to eat, what is to make us think it is even remotely safe for humans to eat?

Medical literature states: It can cause nausea and therapeutic doses can prove fatal to a sensitive person. That's "death." How do you know if you're sensitive or not until you find out the hard way? And what is a therapeutic dose of a poison anyway? Why should we have to worry? Isn't that what the FDA is supposed to be all about?

The **Material Data Sheet** on Sodium Benzoate states:

Ingestion: If swallowed, call a physician immediately.
Induce vomiting
Give oxygen or artificial respiration as needed.

The **Chemical Analysis Sheet** on Sodium Benzoate states:

"Store away from food and beverages."

Even with all the warnings, today it is not kept away from our foods and beverages. In fact, it is found in most of them, including the liquid vitamins that are supposed to "improve your health." Read your vitamin labels. Ask your retailer and distributors of nutritional supplements, to provide a written statement guaranteeing their products are free of stearates, palmitates, stearic acid, food coloring, "natural flavors" meaning MSG, polyethylene glycol, acetate, titanium dioxide, sucrose and any other potentially harmful manufacturing additives and toxic excipients.

The International Pharmaceutical Council of America defines that: "Excipients are substances other than the pharmacologically active ingredients which are included in the manufacturing process or are contained in a finished product. In many products, excipients make up the bulk of the total dosage form."

Many of these excipients carry negative connotations, so the manufacturer choses a euphemistically derived alternative to soften possible undesirable psychological effects such as using the words "glaze" or "natural vegetable coating" in place of SHELLAC, which is made from Shellac Beetles. Even go a step further and ask for full label disclosure listing every component used to produce each product.

Sodium Nitrate and Sodium Nitrite- used to prevent growth of bacteria which causes botulism. Sodium Nitrite adds a pinkish color to foods and is used in lunchmeats, ham, hot dogs, smoked fish and many other meat products. Both, nitrates and nitrites are toxic at only moderate levels. Sodium Nitrate is potentially dangerous to small children, infants and fetuses in pregnant women. Many infants have died from nitrite poisoning as well as many being incapacitated. The government ban on the use of sodium nitrite in fish, is "highly overlooked."

Nitrites convert hemoglobin into methemoglobin which it turn, results in death from the hemoglobin's failure to transport oxygen. Though infants are much more susceptible to nitrates and nitrites than adults, both are still out in many infant foods and formulas.

Both nitrates and nitrites have also been proven highly carcinogenic. Nitrites are transformed into nitrosamines simply by heating or activated by acids in the stomach. These are highly carcinogenic. **Stay away from both!**

CHECK YOUR VITAMINS

Stearates (stearic acid)- better known as "Magnesium Stearate" and "Calcium Stearate" are made by hydrogenating cottonseed or palm oil and are used throughout the supplements industry as machinery lubricants, not health supplements. They are added to raw materials in supplements so production machinery will run at maximum speeds. Over 90% of ALL the vitamins consumed today contain magnesium stearate. Stearic acid inhibits T-cell-dependent, immune responses, or hinders our immune system. In addition, plasma membrane integrity is significantly impaired, leading to loss of cell function and viability. Stearic acid impedes absorption and can lead to liver damage. So much for our taking vitamins to be healthy. If we do, by chance, absorb them, they could kill our liver. Read your labels, thoroughly!

Concentrated magnesium stearate is classified by the Environmental Protection Agency as a hazardous substance and companies that manufacture and transport it must file a Material Safety Data Sheet.

In the EPA data files, Stearic Acid uses are listed as:

"Ammunition dusting powder"

"Paint and varnish dryer"

"Binder and Emulsifier"

The section "Human Health Data" clearly states:

"Inhalation may irritate the respiratory tract."

and

"Acute indigestion, may cause gastroenteritis."

Manufacturers of nutritional supplements push magnesium stearate off to the unsuspecting consumer, as a harmless form of magnesium. Magnesium stearate is the magnesium salt isolated from stearic acid. It is argued that small amount of these substances can do no harm. Why be in there at all?

These hydrogenated oils are meant to speed production machinery up. They do not speed the human machinery up, except maybe towards the toilet or the graveyard. They have nothing to do with health and on the contrary, cause great health hazards. These are hydrogenated, saturated fats, and nowhere on that ingredients label is there an indication of saturated fats to be found.

How much of this substance does it take to cause harm? As much as 5% of the average 1000 mg capsule or tablet is comprised of magnesium stearate. That's 50 mg (milligrams) Let's say you were to take 8 capsules a day. That comes to 250 pills a month or 12,500 milligrams of, unlisted on the label, hydrogenated oils. This is almost half an ounce. In a years' time, that adds up to roughly 6 ounces of hydrogenated oil, that were not listed on the labels, taking just 8 pills on a daily basis. While we are making strides to avoid these toxins in our diets, we are ingesting pounds of them in what we were led to believe to be a product for our health.

Sulphites- used as a preservative from burgers to biscuits, frozen mushrooms and horseradish. Used to make old produce look fresh. Sulphites are banned from MOST foods in the U.S. as they can cause bronchial problems, low blood pressure, tingling and anaphylactic shock. (allergic reaction shock) Avoid at all costs. Especially, if you suffer from bronchial asthma, cardiovascular or respiratory problems and emphysema.

Triphenylmethane Dyes- One of the most common forms of these is light green and another color is "fast green." All are proven carcinogens. They cause cancer! They're FDA approved.

All the above-mentioned additives are "FDA Approved" as safe to be put in our foods and in our mouths. Many are proven carcinogens. Strangely enough, in 1992, Congress passed a law allowing the FDA to be 100% funded by the pharmaceutical companies. Let's try to figure this complicated equation out: Who pays for the FDA testing that still allows carcinogens to be placed in our foods? Who trains our doctors and runs the hospitals that treat all these cancer patients? And who is making all the money? There are over 5,000 more additives that go into our foods, most are unproven safe for human consumption (without ill side effects.) READ YOUR LABELS!

MICROWAVE POPCORN

Uh, oh…I hate to completely rain on the party but…
Did you know: the inside of your microwave popcorn sacks are covered with a chemical that makes the bag oil and heat resistant? They are called "fluorotelomers" and when ingested, the EPA has proven, that the body converts these chemicals into "perfluorooctanoic acid" (PFOA,) a likely carcinogen. Though Fluorotelomers are not initially placed on the popcorn itself, when the super high heat of the microwave hits these oils and artificial buttery flavorings, EPA tests show enough is leached into a single serving to spike the amount of the chemical in your blood. And the buttery flavoring used on that popcorn, called "Diacetyl" is causing bronchiolitis obliterans, "Popcorn Lung" disease. Popping just two bags releases enough residue into your

home to equal the airborne amounts detected in the popcorn factories where this disease is found.

When you open that freshly popped and steaming bag in your face, you've just ingested a sizable amount of these chemicals. EPA tests show 80% of these emissions are released as the bag is opened, not while cooking, and continue at low levels for some minutes after being opened. There have been other incidences in domestic homes, of persons consuming two bags a day, developing this lung disease.

Be aware that Diacetyl is NOT the only chemical in the manufacturing of these flavored popcorn plants that is being examined. Its best to air-pop your popcorn, spray on a little Olive Oil and sprinkle on your favorite "healthy" flavoring.

WATCH OUT FOR THE PLASTIC

"Dude, when are you gonna give us some <u>good</u> news?" In a minute, I promise. But since we're on the topic of chemicals in our foods, there is a huge movement to remove a particular toxic material from our food containers made of plastics.

Phthalates are used to make plastics soft and pliable. Leaching from millions of products such as cosmetics, varnishes, and the coatings of time-released pharmaceuticals, these toxins are absorbed into our blood, urine, saliva, seminal fluids, breast milk and amniotic fluids.

Within food containers and many plastic bottles made of phthalates, there is now another compound called "**Bisphenol**" or (**BPA**.) If you look under your plastic water bottle or other plastic container, you will find a triangle with a number in it. This number represents the times of recycling this plastic has been through. Anything other than the number "1", you do not want to use around food or beverages, especially if they are going to have any heat applied. The higher the number, the more times recycled, and the higher the possibilities for higher amounts of accumulative bisphenol being present.

BPA, an estrogen derivative, is proven to cause hormonal problems in adults as well as hormonal problems and brain defects in children. These chemicals disrupt the endocrine system by imitating the female hormone, estrogen. It is also highly believed to be one of the culprits of obesity, as when given to rats, it causes their insulin levels to soar wildly and crash into a state of resistance, the virtual definition of diabetes.

Marc Goldstein, M.D., Director of the Cornell Institute for Reproductive Medicine notes that: pregnant women are particularly vulnerable. *"Prenatal exposure, even in very low doses, can cause irreversible damage to an unborn baby's reproductive organs."* These chemicals are extremely dangerous to newborns, whose brains, immune systems and gonads are still developing. BPA's have been proven to cause abnormalities in the prostate stem cells, which is the cell implicated in prostate cancer.

Polycarbonate baby bottles are among the products made from this substance. Most being #7, the worst. Many of the clear plastic wrap on foods, contain BPA. Even the plastic liners in the canned goods you deliberately purchased in order to better your health, are made with bisphenol. Heating, freezing or re-using, leaches the toxic chemical from the plastic into the substance contained within. We're eating these plasticizing additives, drinking them, breathing them and absorbing them through our skin on a daily basis.

Bisphenol has been found in the bloodstream of nearly every individual tested. It is best to use glass containers for drinking or storage or find containers that are BPA-FREE. Many nowadays are specifying this right on the container.

I don't want to go off on a total Kevin Trudeau rampage but, isn't it just totally disgusting, the value of the dollar is worth more than a person's health or their life? The original human inhabitants of this earth were created healthy and chemical-free, as were the fruits and vegetables put here to sustain these humans. Is someone trying to say the Creator made all of this WRONG, all of these mistakes, that the human's fruits and vegetables are not complete, are not healthy, are not perfect, are not whole unless they are pumped full of disease-causing, carcinogenic, man-made chemicals? How dare a creator to do such a thing! Or are they saying, "Here little dumb, unsuspecting human, I have a nice, tasty, FDA approved biscuit for you that's going to hook you on all my pills and make me rich beyond my wildest dreams, and I don't care if it kills you?"

Its time to wake up! Its time to start reading labels. You know now what to look for and look out for. And, its time to start writing letters. Don't let them take away your health, your life or the health and lives of your loved ones. You don't need a constitution to stand up for your health, your children's health and their children's, children's health. And thank you, Kevin Trudeau. You are still making a difference!

CHAPTER 8

TREATING THE ORGANIC BODY

Our bodies are made up of 100% organic compounds. We are the grasses that grow wild across the plains. We are the fragrant blossoming fruits of the vine. We are the vegetables of the earth, bathing in the warm sunshine and the gentle rain that caresses their tender flesh. We are the wild flowers radiating in vast rainbows of color sweeping over meadows and valleys, and the wind that choreographs our dances of life, is the very breathe of the Universe that gives us life itself. These are the elements we are. We are the earth. We are Nature's children. We have been created through love and harmony. This is the way our bodies were designed, to work in harmony with one another, in synchronicity, as a "whole." All of our organs and systems work in harmony with one another, in synchronicity, as a whole. They are still individuals, but synergistically, inner-connected as a whole. If one organ begins to fail, the organs on either side must take up the slack.

As they then become overworked, their neighbors must bear the extra burden until the entire body, instead of racing around in synergistic harmony, is now stumbling around on crutches. What was once designed as a flawless and perfectly tuned "system," is now becoming a disconnected pile of individual broken parts and problems. We can't just remove the faulty parts and expect to restore balance and synchronicity. How can you remove parts and expect to make a person "Whole" again?

Blood is your healer. Your blood is visiting every part of your body every several hours. If you have a problem in your knee, your blood is visiting that knee every few hours. What's in your blood will pass through your joints. If that knee receives good digested building materials, you have a very good chance of repairing that knee.

Your blood is also visiting your bowels every few hours. If your eliminative systems are backed up with toxic sludge, your toxic sludge also visits the knee. You can never heal the knee because the blood visits the bowels, the stomach and the liver. The knee can only be as clean as the bowel. Cleaning the bowels cleanses the blood and repairs the knee. In talking of the specific repairing of the knee, we are only treating 5% of the body. We are forgetting that 95% of the patient, was on the other end of the body.

NATURE DOESN'T MAKE MISTAKES

From the time of your birth, your DNA has been programmed for perfection. As we begin and continue adding toxins and toxic waste to the once perfect equation, we are ever pushing the original focal alignment of the body, out of alignment and out of sight. In other words, if we were to take two wheels, lay one on top of the other, we would be representing our DNA's focal point of perfection. Now, if we were to slide the top wheel off to one side, we have caused the wheels to become out of perfect alignment. So far this sounds boring, I realize that. But, stay with me.

Let's call the wheel on the bottom, wheel #1 (representing our body's original DNA programming at the time of birth) and the top wheel, we'll call wheel #2 (representing our body's present condition) As toxins are introduced to the body, not expelled frequently enough and continue to accumulate, they are continually pushing wheel #2 out of alignment with wheel #1. We now begin operating away from the ultimate state of perfection. Instead of rolling down the road in total harmony and ease, our wheels are now trying to roll separate ways and force the other to follow. They can't even travel the simple path of a straight line without a struggle. Our body must now begin to make adjustments and compensations for the out-of-balance state it is now forced to function within.

Systems will begin to break down and organs will fail. This forces the healthier organs to take up the slack for their faltering neighbor organ and if their neighbor isn't restored back to health, they themselves' eventually begin to break down, due to the extra workload placed upon them.

Just as drugs suppress symptoms, organs taking up the slack for deficient organs will assimilate a symptom-suppressing type action. It is a temporary fix that is causing everything to eventually break down. This is primarily and temporarily covering up for their belabored neighbor, similar to one brother covering for another, so mom and dad won't find out, at least for a while. But, it can't continue forever. There is an end to this bumpy road. As always, all good things must come to an end and the truth will surface.

Our body begins to show signs of breaking down. In the case of the immune system, we may begin developing more frequent head colds that begin turning into chest colds, then bronchitis, becoming resistant to antibiotics, eventually developing into pneumonia and ending in emphysema, lung cancer or death.

The body can only hold out for so long until the ammunition runs out and the army surrenders to the constant bombardment of toxins and putrefied wastes, without the support of the nutritional infantry and your immune system has long gone laid down their weapons and headed for the hills.

THE HEART OF THE PROBLEM
Treating the Organic

Here is a true example of what happens when the body becomes toxic and organs begin to fail as the body's natural balance is lost.

Barney Clark, received a heart transplant and survived nearly a year. But, within a six-month period, he developed pneumonia. (Remember, the lungs are part of the elimination channels.) He recovered from the pneumonia but three months later, developed trouble in another one of the eliminative channels, the kidneys;. He died three months later of "Bowel Toxemia."

The heart was the sole focus of the operation. They had completely overlooked the condition of the other 95% of the patient's body. It was not ready to handle a new heart. He was not treated "as a whole."

We can't just go on treating symptoms. There's a whole lotta human on the other end of that symptom. We must be treated as a "whole."

Test question: How many blood pressure pills does it take to cure a high blood pressure problem? The answer is NONE.

Ever seen it done?

How many people have you heard of being cured of "High Blood Pressure" from taking blood pressure medicine? I will guess the answer to be, NO ONE. If they stop taking the pills, does the blood pressure not start rising right back up? That doesn't sound like much of a cure.

If you broke the chemistry down in your blood pressure medicine, you will find a lot of strange words and none of which were ever present in your original body chemistry at birth. Are we again, trying to say, "Nature, you made a mistake and forgot to put some of these needed chemicals in our chemistry make-up?" Or, is Nature saying, you put something in there that wasn't supposed to be in there and YOU made a BIG mistake, i.e., salt, trans-saturated fats, mold, yeast, fungus, alcohol, GMO foods, drugs, medicines and a barrage of other toxic wastes?

We are a totally organic body made from the perfect elemental compounds of the earth. Again, Nature doesn't make mistakes. When we go mixing man-made pharmaceutical chemicals, made from coal-tar and petroleum bases, we are doing nothing more than mixing water and oil (dirty water and over-cooked oils) and expecting a harmonious compatibility. Can't be done! We are poisoning the system. We are destroying nature's perfect creation.

There's a very old book that most people in our country own and many read on a daily basis. It's a very popular book. It not only tells one how to act, it also tells one how to eat. It also says, "Your body is your temple." If we were talking about a physical building, would you dump a barrel of garbage in the middle of the floor, or pour raw sewage in the middle of the room and leave it there? Would you stomp and wallow around in grease, tracking it all through the rest of your temple? Would you disgrace and disrespect this temple in such a manner? Then why do we keep doing it to our spiritual temple, our bodies? This IS the house of your spirit, at least for the time being, and you only get one. Take care of it!

Some people talk about stem-cell research and cloning people or body parts and how wrong it is to be pretending we are God, to alter God's creation, his perfect creation. Well, what do you think you are doing when you pop that handful of prescription pills in your face? These synthetic, <u>man-made</u>, body-altering compounds that synthetically alter the natural physiological functions of your God-made body?

We take a pill to control the heart, a pill to thin our blood, a pill to control our sugar, one to control our cholesterol, a pill for depression, a pill to sleep, a pill to wake up, a pill to "get it up" and another to perk us up. We take uppers to get us up out of bed and downers to bring us off the ceiling. We take a pill to relieve, a pill to conceive, a pill for a cough, a pill for a sneeze, a pill to breathe and give our dogs one for fleas! Do you not call that synthetically altering the perfect creation, just a bit? Destroying the perfect creation of the Creator who created this perfected temple masterpiece to begin with? Would you trash a multi-million dollar "Picasso"? Each one of our bodies is worth much more than any Picasso, Rembrandt, Michael Angelo or Leonardo Da Vince. When do we invent the pill to wake us all up and restore common sense? This out-of-control pharmaceutical epidemic is brain-washing everyone into half-synthetic, zombie/sheeple, who are not even functioning by their own natural abilities. It's also killing helplessly trusting, unaware and innocent people by the tune of:

"**100,000+** in 2017, who died as a result of prescription drugs. And this was just from pharmaceutical overdoses."

This doesn't count the fatal side effects of the drugs, as mentioned in most of their ads. They won't release that number. But you can bet it nearly double the first one, or more. Why is someone not going to jail over this?

GET TO THE ROOT OF THE PROBLEM

If you have "High Cholesterol" you aren't deficient in Lipitor, you have eaten too much animal meat, cheese and dairy, the only source of cholesterol on the planet, except for the cholesterol produced by the liver. Ever see a hunk of fat hanging from a vegetable or a piece of fruit? No. You can only acquire outside cholesterol from animal flesh., meats and animal by-products.

Then there's that bunch of bowel movement they try to suck you in with about getting cholesterol from your " sweet Auntie Jane" or good ol' "Uncle Fred." Sorry, the only way you're ever gonna get cholesterol from these folks is if you eat them.
I'll leave the method of preparation up to you. Don't have a recipe for "poached Grannie."

So, how does one stop one's cholesterol from rising? Take a pill? No. Stop eating from the source.

What's causing your High Blood Pressure? Unless you have an actual heart defect, salt, grease, toxic buildup, animal fats and excess weight.

Did you know that: for every ten pounds of fat you put on, your body has to make 3 to 5 thousand miles of capillaries to supply blood to that fat or gangrene will set in?

Think of how much extra burden that places on the heart. Then, add the veins and the arteries that are plugging up from hydrogenated, trans-fats and free radical damage. What happens to these extra capillaries when we lose the weight? The body just simply re-absorbs them. Isn't Nature amazing?

Let's say you had a chair in the middle of your bedroom floor, right smack in the middle of the path to the toilet. You get up in the middle of the night for your first trip to relieve yourself and you stub your toe. "Damn, that hurt!" So, you stumble to the medicine cabinet, grab a pain pill, hobble into the kitchen for a glass of water, because you just knocked the bathroom glass off the counter, trying to find the light switch. So you go lie in bed until the throbbing quits. Then, Nature calls again. You get up, stub the same damn toe again, on the same damn chair in the middle of the floor. Now, the last dose of pain medicine isn't touching the excruciating pain shooting up your leg to the middle of your brain. So, we grab a stronger version.

Now, would you continue to keep stubbing your toe, night after night and taking stronger and stronger medicine, when you could cure the problem by simply removing the chair? Why not get right to the root of your illness, remove the symptoms by removing or CURING the cause?

TREATMENTS FOR MORE COMMAN ILLNESES

These are proven protocols I have use for many years will excellent success. These are not "symptom-suppressors" These treatments get to the ROOT CAUSE of the illness.

ADDICTION

Whether it's an addiction to chocolate or an addiction to alcohol, sleeping pills, cigarettes or cocaine, the mechanisms of chemical addictions all work the same. There are residues or "chemical markers" released into the bloodstream from the addictive substance. As long as these markers are detected in adequate supply within the bloodstream, the body has no adverse reactions. But when the markers drop below the level the body has grown accustomed to, the body will react in whatever way necessary to get its fix. This can be experienced as jitters, cramps, headaches, contraction from minimal to quite violent, depending on the severity needed to get a response.

The usual negative results experienced by detox clinics and hospitals is due to the fact of trying to replace one drug with another, while never attempting to remove the addictive substance to start with. It's still there. It is going to cause reactions. It is going to cause misery.

The secret to the successful detoxification of such a problem is to flush the toxins from the body quickly, before they have a chance to react.

At our facility we have witnessed full blown cocaine addicts, alcoholics, heroin addicts, opioid addicts all become free of the addictive substance in three days with absolutely no side effects; no DT's, no shakes, no vomiting, no anything but successful results.. The following is the standard protocol used in every such case.

1. Full Body Detox
2. Daily D-Oxygen Bath treatments.

After that, addictive substance no longer has any effect on the patient. We have had tramadol addicts say the drugs seemed to be pulled out of their body in the first hour of the D-Oxy Bath alone. Numerous patients would ask, "When am I going to have the DT's?" It just doesn't happen with this method.

ADRENAL REPAIR

The Adrenals sit atop each kidney. They are your "fight or flight" mechanisms. If you are endangered, stressed or upset, your adrenals, sense trouble and begin to pump "adrenaline," a neurotransmitter, and "Cortisol," a steroid hormone, are released into the system.

Adrenaline, or epinephrine, and cortisol, or hydrocortisone, are stress hormones. Though both chemicals are stress hormones, adrenaline and cortisol play different biochemical roles. Adrenaline primarily binds to receptors on the heart and heart vessels. This increases heart rate, force of muscle contraction and respiration. Cortisol binds to receptors on the fat cells, liver and pancreas, which increases glucose levels available for muscles to use. It also temporarily inhibits other systems of the body, including digestion, growth, reproduction and the immune system. It has been proven that persons with sleep deprivation due to adrenal failure, have a cortisol level 85% higher than the normal healthy level. You MUST lower the cortisol level to correct this problem.

COMPLETE SYSTEMS DETOX- Liver/Gallbladder, Intestines, Kidneys, Tissues
This sets the stage for repair to begin.

1, **Ashwagandha**- Ashwagandha (*Withania somnifera*) is a traditional adaptogenic Ayurvedic herb used mainly for anxiety. It belongs to a select group of herbs referred to as *adaptogens*, natural remedies that counter the physical and mental effects of stress. Adaptogens are neither stimulating nor sedating but bring the body into a state of balance known as homeostasis.

2. Rhodiola rosea- is another adaptogenic herb used in traditional Chinese medicine to increase vigor and stamina. It reduces cortisol and increases resilience to stress but is slightly energizing rather than sedating. This makes it a good choice if you are both stressed and fatigued. It's been found to alleviate depression symptoms rapidly, even faster than antidepressant medications. It also increases dopamine, serotonin, and nor-epinephrine — brain chemicals that have an appreciable impact on mood.

3. Cordyceps-(*Cordyceps sinensis*) is a fungus used in traditional Chinese medicine mainly to increase stamina and promote longevity. You won't find cordyceps growing in the woods though; this fungus grows on the backs of caterpillars!
Cordyceps has been found to improve physical performance and <u>lower cortisol levels</u>; however, it also increases two shorter-lived and less damaging stress hormones, epinephrine and nor-epinephrine

4. Phosphatidylserine- is a fat that naturally occurs in high concentrations in the brain and nervous system. PS reduces the effects of both physical and mental stress by keeping cortisol levels down. Phosphatidylserine is an outstanding brain supplement in its own right.

5. L-Theanine- is an amino acid found almost exclusively in black, green, white, and Oolong tea. It is widely regarded for inducing a state of "calm attentiveness." Promotes better sleep, reduces caffeine jitters, improves mood, better cognition.
For <u>cortisol reduction, L-Theanine is tops</u> .

It would be hard to consume this much L-Theanine from tea which generally has 25 mg per cup, but you can easily get a 200 mg dose with an L-Theanine supplement.

Note: Any substance that stimulates; coffee, Monster Drinks, Red Bull, Soda, etc. will activate the Adrenals.
Stress also activates the adrenals.
With continued activation, the adrenals become overworked and begin "burnout."
This elevates the Cortisol levels in the blood resulting in inability to sleep or even think clearly.
Remove as much of the stress irritant as possible.
Clean up the diet from fast foods, fried foods, processed sugars, energy drinks and polluted foods.

Meditate and stay calm…Grasshopper.

ALLERGIES

Note: No one should have an allergy to anything organic.
As for allergies, **this is why you have them**:

The main part of the immune system sits upon the intestinal tract. It scans every molecule of food that passes from the stomach to the small intestine. Each molecule is marked "accepted" or "rejected."
Did you know: 75% of your immune system sits on top of your digestive system, as well as does 60% of you lymph nodes.

When a person continually eats bad foods that continually is having to be rejected by the immune guards, the immune system becomes "Hyper-Active." With continuation of these eating habits one begins to develop holes in the intestinal tract. This is referred to as "Leaky Gut Syndrome." this condition is further added to by alcohol and many medicines such as the common aspirin, pain killers and antacids, along with coffee, sodas, etc.
Through these holes, unchecked and unprocessed proteins are allowed to escape into the bloodstream.

The body's defense system, already being hyper-active and on high alert, recognizes these intruders and begins creating antigens to combat these enemies. Before long, the neighbor's cat can walk across the yard and you go into an allergy attack because the immune system is hyper-active. Now, you didn't eat this cat, or even pet it, but the Hyper-Active immune system says you are now allergic to it.

To address allergies, you must repair the leaky gut caused from drugs, acidic foods such as fried and acidic drinks like coffee, soda, alcohol, energy drinks and black teas, artificial sweeteners, antibiotics. This should take 30-60 days from end of Detox.

This is what to do:

1. Remove all body toxins
2. Change the eating habits to avoid fried foods, acidic drinks, alcoholic beverages, processed sugars, preservatives, artificial sweeteners and medicines, specifically pain suppressors like aspirins or stronger.
3. **Take these following supplements:**

1. L-Glutamine is an amino acid that is fundamental to the well-being of the digestive and immune systems. Glutamine is great for repairing damage to the gut, helping the gut lining to regrow and repair, undoing the damage caused by leaky gut, and reducing sugar cravings. I recommend 3-5 grams a day.

2. Digestive Enzymes Digestive enzymes are plant or microbial-based supplements that support the breakdown, absorption, and utilization of macronutrients. Taken with meals, they work with the body's own reduced supply of enzymes to achieve maximum digestion and support intestinal repair mechanisms.

3. Betaine Hydrochloric Acid (HCL) Betaine hydrochloride (HCL) promotes optimal gastric acidity for support of protein digestion and absorption of minerals and other nutrients such as vitamin B12. There is a simple at home test you can do to see if you have low stomach acid and are in need of HCL replacement. Begin to eat a meal and ⅓ of the way into your meal take 650 mg of HCL and then finish your meal. If you experience heartburn, you have sufficient levels of HCL. If you do not experience any burning sensation in your upper abdomen, then you likely would benefit from HCL at each meal.

4. Slippery Elm It might have kind of a strange name, but slippery elm has been used as an effective gut healer for centuries in the United States. This supplement both contains mucilage and stimulates nerve endings in the body's intestinal tract to increase natural mucus secretion, which is an instrumental part of the stomach's protective lining and helps combat ulcers and excessive acidity in the digestive system. It also contains important antioxidants that help relieve inflammatory bowel symptoms.

5. De-glycyrrhizinated Licorice (DGL) DGL is an herb that has been used for over 3,000 years in the treatment of digestive issues including ulcers and indigestion. It's made from whole licorice, but the manufacturing process includes the removal of glycyrrhizin, which can cause an elevation in blood pressure. DGL supports the body's natural processes for maintaining the mucosal lining of the stomach and duodenum.

6. Marshmallow Root Marshmallow root is a multipurpose supplement that can be used for respiratory or digestive relief. Like slippery elm, it contains a high mucilage content. It eases the inflammation in the stomach lining, heals ulcers, and treats both diarrhea and constipation by creating a protective lining on the digestive tract.

7. Caprylic Acid, also known as octanoic acid, is a naturally occurring fatty acid that comes from coconut oil. Calcium and magnesium caprylates act as buffers and may also help slow the dispersion and release of caprylic acid to support its activity throughout the gastrointestinal tract. Caprylic acid is known for its antiviral and antifungal activity. For those who feel that you may be suffering from Candida or yeast overgrowth this is a safe, effective and natural way to treat Candida.

The Leaky Gut Diet and 5 Healing Foods

If you suffer from leaky gut syndrome, you're overdue to consider adopting a **leaky gut diet**. Here are the five foods and supplements to heal your leaky gut.

#1 Bone Broth – broth contains collagen and the amino acids proline and glycine that can help heal your damaged cell walls. I've had many of my patients do a bone broth fast for three days to help heal leaky gut and cure autoimmune disease.

#2 Raw Cultured Dairy – contains both probiotics and SCFA's that can help heal the gut. Pastured **kefir**, yogurt, amazia, butter and raw cheese are some of the best.

#3 Fermented Vegetables – contain organic acids that balance intestinal pH and probiotics to support the gut. Sauerkraut, kimchi and kvass are excellent sources or make your own.

#4 Coconut Products – all **coconut** products are especially good for your gut. The MCFA's in coconut are easier to digest than other fats so they work well for leaky gut. Also, coconut kefir contains probiotics that support your digestive system.

#5 Sprouted Seeds – chia seeds, flaxseeds and **hemp seeds** that have been sprouted are great sources of fiber that can help support the growth of beneficial bacteria. But if you have severe leaky gut, you may need to start out getting your fiber from steamed vegetables and fruit.

Also, consuming foods that have omega-3 fats are beneficial — **anti-inflammatory foods** like grass-fed beef, lamb and wild-caught fish like salmon.

ALZHEIMERS/DEMENTIA PROTOCOL

Begin Protocol with Castle in the Clouds':
Complete Detox Program

This will assure the majority of toxins and cellular debris are removed, enhancing the effectiveness of any protocol. Crucial for combating chronic illnesses.

Omni-Immune- (15 drops 2 x day) start w/6 drops and work up to max dosage Cleans arteries, veins and capillaries)

READ ALL OMNI-IMMUNE DIRECTIONS THOROUGHLY BEFORE ADMINISTERING!!!
(Available ONLY from Castle in the Clouds)

The following supplements can be found on Amazon.com or Vitacost.com

Lipo-Spheric Glutathione (Liv-On Labs or Readi-Sorb) I suggest the latter product.
"Removes most dementia and Alzheimer's symptoms almost immediately.
Start with 3x's the recommended dose for the first 3 days, then follow box instructions.

NADH w/ATP (may have to buy ATP separately)" Source Natural Sublinguals" or "Now" brand (Brain stimulant)

ATP- "Pro Health Ultra ATP+ (Lights brain on fire) amazing. ATP works synergistically with NADH (must use both to work)

Ultra-Liquid Zeolite w/DHQ (Detoxes heavy metal

Astaxanthin- "Bio-Astin" brand 12mg time release (Rebuilds Brain and Heart)

Super Neurogen DHA – "Genestra" brand (Made from Algae, not Fish Oil) Brain function enhancer

Intra-Max Liquid Vit/Min (Can be purchased from Castle in the Clouds) 415 Bio-Available nutrients from "Live" cultures. In blood 100% in 15 minutes. Contains ALL vitamins, minerals, pro-biotics, amino-acids, 70 plant extracts. Incredible.

Electrolyte Supplement (Liquid, if possible) Coconut water is excellent. But you may need a more concentrated dose than it can supply.

Magnesium L-Threonate- protects against cognitive decline.

L-Theanine "for anxiety" If depressed, use **L-Tryptophan** We suggest "Doctors Best" brand

Dosage:
Take 3x's recommended dosage for one or two days, then follow instructions.

Melatonin- 10 mg minimum at night (For sleep aid)
Magnesium- 400-800 mg. before bed as a sleep aid. Works wonders.

ANXIETY
(PANIC ATTACKS)

Affects women twice as much as men. Due to the hormonal bio-rhythm charts of women.

The base cause can be food allergy reaction (corn, wheat, cow's milk, etc.) or a severe hypoglycemic reaction.
If you recall: Emotions are held in the "gut" as well as your digestive system and the 75% of you immune system. It ALL works together.

Treatment:
Full Body Detox
Supplementation (after cleansing):
Chromium and Vanadium- 200-300 mcg a day
B6- 100 mg a day
B3- 450 mg a day (time released)

B1, B2 and B5- 50 mg a day
L-Tryptophan- 10 grams until attack ceases
Calcium- 2000 mg a day
Magnesium- 800 mg per day
Betaine HCI 100-250 mg until attack ceases
Valerian can be of value
Avoid caffeine and processed sugar, concentrated fruit juices, candy, sodas.

ARTHRITIS

Let's break down and analyze physical body parts in a simplistic manner. Your joints have been diagnosed as having arthritis. Any word ending in "itis" means irritated. Your joints feel painful, not because they are old, but because they have gritty, grinding toxic deposits accumulated and causing inflammation and sometimes, great pain.

If you were to take your ball-joint of your car, pour some sand in, before long, that sand will start to affect the performance of the joint and eventually it would need replacing, because the sand, grit or gravel, the irritant was not removed. If your car were alive and had feeling sensors, it would be in great pain and crying out for help. In a sense, that's exactly what it does when it begins to shake and shimmy. Its saying, "you probably waited too long." And now it must be replaced. Don't wait 'til then to fix your body. Do it before it cries for help.

If you put acid or another corrosive material on steel, it begins to deteriorate. Same thing goes for hip replacements. Too much acidic and toxic waste laid against the hip and its sockets for too long a time and now the erosion and corrosion have overtaken the once healthy body part and neglect has taken its traumatic toll. We now have the "end-point of acid saturation," or death to that body part.

After a thorough cleaning of the bowels and liver, a wonderful and effective way to rid yourself of acid and arthritic symptoms, I suggest the use of these three items: Raw goat milk, Black Mission Figs and Concentrated Goat Whey Protein. (Capra Goat whey is my preference.) It is VERY alkalizing. Color therapy as well as Baking Soda Baths: 1 box in hot bath for 20 minutes, may also be very beneficial. Periodic repetition of the Master Cleanse to further remove debris and accumulative acids from the joints and tissue.

AUTISM

We have seen incredible results with this simple protocol. We have witnessed, wheel-chaired Autistic children, in 6 days, jump on a bed. This is NOT an uncommon result.

Autism is brought on by a deposition of heavy metals. The first step in reversing the damage and removal of debris is the Castle in the Clouds' Complete Body Detoxification System. We have also discovered children deficient in Glutathione are unable to process protein and are more susceptible to Autism.

1 Upon completion of the **detox program**:
2 **Abstain from** ALL

grains	food coloring
dairy	preservatives

        corn   fried foods and trans-fats
        gluten   processed sugar
        GMO foods   hydrogenated oils

3 **A diet** of totally organic foods are crucial at this point

4 Further detoxification will continue with the following
supplemental regimen:

Lipo-Somal Glutathione (Lipo-Spheric)
Ultra Liquid Zeolite w/DHQ
NADH with ATP (Adenosine tri-phosphate)
Ionic Magnesium

This is the end of Stage I. Continued cleansing and healthy
nutritional support will result in continued improvements.

AUTO IMMUNE DISEASES

Autoimmune diseases, specifically, now affect 24 million
people and include rheumatoid arthritis, lupus, multiple sclerosis,
thyroid disease, inflammatory bowel disease, and more.

One huge culprit in the causation and advancement of many
Auto-Immune illness is **"GLUTEN."**

Gluten can, and many times mimic certain specific
antagonistic proteins in the body. This in turn stimulates an
"auto-immuno" response. The immune system not only
recognizes the newly found "mimic proteins," but also mistake
the original copied proteins as intruders as well and therefore
begins its mission of attacking and removing of ALL like
proteins. Hence, the body begins attacking its own tissues,
resulting in a vicious circling battle of immune system vs itself.
If left unchecked, develops into a full blown "Autoimmune"
disorder.

These proteins show up as antagonistic markers in various
places in the body from brain to lungs to digestive system. If an
abundance of these markers are detected in any certain part of the
body, GLUTEN can and predominantly WILL react and very
likely, if left unchecked, stimulate an immuno-response and so
also the beginning of an "Autoimmune Disease."

Heart disease, Alzheimer's, lung diseases and many neurological diseases have been linked to gluten. With the ability to mimic specific proteins in the body, these intruders go unnoticed for a period of time, until the immune system discovers they are actually not what they appeared to be. Then it begins the destruction and removal of these unchecked proteins.

Suddenly, the immune system also discovers, these proteins look almost exactly like the ones in the brain, or the heart, or the lungs. We'd better get rid of them too. Hence, your immune system begins its extraction of the healthy proteins that were supposed to be in your brain, or your heart or wherever. Now, you have a full-scaled war going on inside your body between your body's own personal defense system and itself. The defense system is trying to overthrow its leader.

Gluten may also show up as ingredients in barley malt, chicken broth, malt vinegar, some salad dressings, veggie burgers (if not specified gluten-free), and soy sauce. The protein may even hide in many common seasonings and spice mixes.

Leaky Gut Syndrome is another leading culprit in the line of auto-immune triggers. Unprocessed proteins are leached into the bloodstream via perforations in the gut from over-usage of aspirin and other pain medications, acidic beverages and other intestinal lining irritants. The leaky gut protocol is covered in its own section of this book

Toxins- Many times and most times an autoimmune response is triggered by a saturation of toxic, accumulated-waste not being properly evacuated on a regular basis. Once the saturation point peaks, the immune system has nowhere to go but on the defense, attacking all that gets in its way. The immune system's number one primary job is cleaning house, not repairing. For it knows, if everything is kept clean there will be nothing to repair. A clean house is a healthy house.

Note: To treat and eradicate ANY autoimmune disease, you must first remove the sludge, the toxic accumulations, the medication residues, chemical residues and waste from the liver, the digestive system, the tissues and the blood. Until then, you will

NEVER succeed in truly eradicating an autoimmune disease. Its "Dis - Ease" Your body isn't responding this way because its happy. It is lashing out. It is telling you, "Hey...need some help in here!" Was it not working fine before you acquired this notification? So, put it back the way it was before. Yes, it IS that simple!

Step 1 Full Body Detox (To the max and by the book. No
      exceptions.)

Step 2 Replenish the body with the 90 nutrient building blocks it
      MUST have to heal.

Step 3 Supplement the immune system with extra support:

    L-Lysine- 1000-1200 mg 3x's a day

    Vitamin C- 10,000 mg 1-3x's a day (Lipo-Spheric, is best)

    Omni-Immune- work up to 15 drops 1 or 2x's a day
        (Supports immune and kills pathogens)

    Immune System Support Mushrooms- double or triple
        the dosage on the bottle to build a
        reserve. Then continue taking as
        suggested on the bottle.

    Intra-Max- Liquid vit./min. supplement. 415 nutrients.
        Essential for providing the building
        blocks for "healthy cells that work."

    Brazilian Mushrooms- (Acarigus Blazai) will triple your
        NK (natural killer) cells in 48 hours

    Liquid Chlorophyll- Blood builder, oxygenator and blood
        cleanser.

    Ultra-Liquid Zeolite w/DHQ- removes heavy metals

Step 4 Alkalize the whole system with 80/20 eating regime and
      alkaline water

Step 5 High-Oxygen Therapy is very beneficial especially in
      advanced and stubborn conditions.

Step 6 Rife Treatments if dealing with microbes or pathogens, in
      addition to the Omni-Immune.

CONGESTIVE HEART FAILURE

Always, start with a **Full Body Detox**, unless the person is in a weakened condition.

Hawthorne Berry

If your response to CoQ10 is insufficient, the next step is to add hawthorn berry (Crataegus supp.)as a congestive heart failure treatment. I've used it extensively, particularly in patients sensitive to digoxin. (a medication used for a-fib)

Hawthorn berry can increase the action of digoxin, making it possible to decrease the dose of digoxin, thereby avoiding or lessening digoxin-related side effects.

In fact, some patients with mild congestive heart failure get significant relief with hawthorn berry alone, an effect supported by double-blind studies in Europe. The German government recognizes hawthorn berries as an approved heart medicine.

Hawthorn improves the heart's ability to metabolize energy and utilize oxygen, and the berry's extracts contain flavonoids that increase the heart muscle's force of contraction.

Hawthorn berries also normalize irregular heartbeats, help lower blood pressure and enhance circulation by dilating the arteries.

Aim for 500–1500 mg daily or take as a tincture in water three times daily. For prevention, I recommend drinking hawthorn berry tea, which you can make by pouring boiling water over a cup of berries and letting them steep for 15 minutes.

L-carnitine and L-arginine Amino Acids- increases energy available to the heart muscle cells of congestive heart failure patients by supporting free fatty acid metabolism. Aim for **500 mg twice daily.**

L-arginine- is another amino acid. It improves blood flow to the heart by stimulating endothelial cell releasing factor (ECRF), thereby inhibiting a chain of complex reactions that might otherwise cause plaque to form in the arteries and stifle blood flow to the heart. **Use 2–4 grams before bedtime**.

Levodopa (L-dopa)- In stubborn, severe cases of congestive heart failure, I turn to Levodopa (L-dopa). It's the natural counterpart of an intravenous drug called Dobutamine.

When congestive heart failure approaches terminal stages, cardiologists sometimes opt to administer Dobutamine, although they must hospitalize the patient for half a day in order to closely monitor the individual for dose-related adverse reactions.

Many patients experience an increase in heart muscle strength with this once-weekly treatment, improving the effectiveness of their heart's pumping action.

Like Dobutamine, Levodopa is converted to dopamine in the body and can have similar beneficial effects on the weakened heart, but it can be taken orally.

Vitamin B-6 promotes the conversion of L-dopa to dopamine and should therefore be taken along with the L-dopa to maximize the beneficial heart effects.

L-dopa dosages need to be determined and carefully adjusted for each patient, so you'll need to work with an alternative-minded physician for this treatment. Side effects can include rhythmic muscular twitches, heart palpitations, lightheadedness, nausea and vomiting.

Lily of the Valley and Foxglove-For edema in legs and /or belly. **English Hawthorne:** is useful in regulating heart rhythm.

Respect Your Body

The whole point here is to give your heart, and your quality of life, the best possible chance for improvement. For this to happen, it's critical that you and your physician respect the uniqueness of your body and of your particular heart condition—

every patient is different.

CANCER

This ailment has been skipped deliberately. Due to the extensiveness of the information involved, it has been designated its own separate chapter following the ailment protocols.

CROHN'S, IRRITABLE BOWEL AND DIVERTICULITIS

Crohn's Disease, irritable bowel syndrome, diverticulitis are the end results of toxic sludge not being properly eliminated. It builds up a toxic dam, forcing great pressure on the colon and intestinal walls. The body's defense against toxic waste is mucous. So, mucous is now deposited over the entire digestive tract, smothering the small intestinal villi hair, that lines the intestinal walls and filters nutrients out of the food passing by.

With a thick coat of mucous smashing them flat, similar to ice in grass, the food is no longer filtered by these hairs and the food goes right into the river without any nutritional gain for your poor, already deprived body. The result, diarrhea.

Pressure continues to build up in the colon, from the over-accumulation of mucous. The walls of the intestines and colon begin to press outward, causing stress and weakening. We begin to develop pockets or "diverticula" in the tract walls. Constipation develops. A continued barrage of toxins and mucous force more pressure until the dam ruptures. In the section of this book under curing the human body, I will show you how to rid yourself of this ailment and all others, if you are willing to take charge of your health.

In the case of Crohn's Disease, it is an advanced condition of IBS (Irritable Bowel Syndrome).

- Its causation is an obliterated intestinal tract due to inherent weakness and poor dietary habits
- resulting in a complete breakdown of the digestive system. To combat this condition, the medical world arms themselves with two main medicines, both admittedly cause liver damage and cancer with very little to no results in alleviating this condition whatsoever.

NOTE: It's important not to confuse an inflammatory bowel disease (IBD) like Crohn's disease or ulcerative colitis with irritable bowel syndrome (IBS). IBS is a disorder that affects the muscle contractions of the bowel and is not characterized by intestinal inflammation, nor is it a chronic disease.

There has to be a determined and complete change in dietary habits following an intense detoxification and removal of accumulated fecal matter and toxic wastes. Thereafter, will follow certain foods to avoid, as well as foods to eat and supplements to aid in repairing and rebuilding of the intestinal tract.

We have had articles written about our success with Crohn's disease at our facility. We have completely reversed these conditions using cleansing along with supplementation, combined with a strict eating regime to rebuild intestinal integrity while closing up non-healing, gaping wounds in the colon.

Step One: Cleanses
 Full Body Detox (crucial)
1. Liver-Gallbladder
2. Intestinal Cleanse
3. Kidney/Tissue Cleanse

Following the cleanses, you will begin the eating regime and repair protocols.

FOOD GROUPS TO AVOID

GMO (Genetically Modified Foods)

- Gluten
- Corn
- Soy
- Commercial dairy
- Processed foods
- Refined sugar
- Refined oils
- Additives
- Un-soaked & unsprouted nuts, seeds, and legumes
- Preservatives
- Dyes
  Gluten mimics certain body tissues and can spark an immuno-response, resulting in the body's immune system overreacting, creating an auto-immune disease wherein the immune system is tricked into attacking the body's tissues.

STAY WAY FROM **ALL** ALCOHOL AND TOBACCO PRODUCTS

FOODS THAT FIGHT AND PREVENT INFLAMMATION

Blueberries	Turmeric	Tomatoes	Whole Grains	Apples
Coconut Oil	Raw Oats	Beets	Chia Seeds	Eggs
Nuts	Raw Honey	Ginger	Broccoli	Pineapple
Garlic	White Tuna	Miso	Green Tea	Black Beans
Spinach	Kamut	Rosemary		

Fermented Veggies (These are exceptionally beneficial)
Wild Salmon   Extra-Virgin Olive Oil   Yogurt   Bone Broth

"THE 4 R'S REGIMINE"|

Step 1: Remove

In this first step we remove the offending foods and toxins from your diet that could be acting as stressors on your system. This means caffeine, alcohol, processed foods, bad fats, and any other foods you think may be causing issues, like gluten and dairy. All of these irritate the gut in some form and create an inflammatory response.

Step 2: Repair

The next step is to begin to repair the gut and heal the damaged intestinal lining. You do this by consuming an unprocessed diet and giving your body time to rest by providing it with substances that are known to heal the gut, like L-glutamine, omega-3 fatty acids, zinc, antioxidants (in the form of vitamins A, C, and E), quercetin, aloe vera, and turmeric.

Step 3: Restore

This involves the restoration of your gut's optimal bacterial flora population. This is done with the introduction of probiotics like *Lactobacillus acidophilus* and *Bifidobacterium lactis*. A probiotic is a good bacteria and is ingested to help reinforce and maintain a healthy gastrointestinal tract and to help fight illness. In general a healthy lower intestinal tract should contain around 85% good bacteria. This helps to combat any overgrowth of bad bacteria. Unfortunately in most people these percentages are skewed, and this allows for the gut health to drastically decline. The human gut is home to bad bacteria like salmonella and clostridium, which is fine as long as they are kept in order and don't get out of control. Stay alkaline.

Step 4: Replace

This involves getting your bile salts, digestive enzymes, and hydrochloric acid levels to optimal levels to maintain and promote healthy digestion. This can be done by supplementing with digestive enzymes and organic salt to help make sure you have enough hydrochloric acid. One of the BEST ways to repair and replace it with Cultured Vegetables.
These are fermented, similar to sauerkraut and are loaded with bacterial cultures crucial in rebuilding and healing of the digestive tract. The starter cultures a direction can be purchased at " www.bodyecology.com

Supplementation:
1. L-Glutamine is an amino acid that is fundamental to the well-

being of the digestive and immune systems. Glutamine is great for repairing damage to the gut, helping the gut lining to regrow and repair, undoing the damage caused by leaky gut, and reducing sugar cravings.
Dosage: 3-5 grams a day. (3,000-5000 mg)

2. Digestive Enzymes- are plant or microbial-based supplements that support the breakdown, absorption, and utilization of macronutrients. Taken with meals, they work with the body's own reduced supply of enzymes to achieve maximum digestion and support intestinal repair mechanisms.
Dosage: 1-2 capsules with every meal.

3. Betaine Hydrochloric Acid (HCL)- promotes optimal gastric acidity for support of protein digestion and absorption of minerals and other nutrients such as vitamin B12. There is simple at home test you can do to see if you have low stomach acid and are in need of HCL replacement. Begin to eat a meal and ⅓ of the way into your meal take 650 mg of HCL and then finish your meal. If you experience heartburn, you have sufficient levels of HCL. If you do not experience any burning sensation in your upper abdomen, then you likely would benefit from HCL at each meal.
Dosage: 2 capsules with every meal;

4. Slippery Elm- might have kind of a strange name, but slippery elm has been used as an effective gut healer for centuries in the United States. This supplement both contains mucilage and stimulates nerve endings in the body's intestinal tract to increase natural mucus secretion, which is an instrumental part of the stomach's protective lining and helps combat ulcers and excessive acidity in the digestive system. It also contains important antioxidants that help relieve inflammatory bowel symptoms.
Dosage: 100 mg 3x's day

5. Deglycyrrhizinated Licorice (DGL)- DGL is an herb that has been used for over 3,000 years in the treatment of digestive issues including ulcers and indigestion. It's made from whole licorice, but the manufacturing process includes the removal of glycyrrhizin, which can cause an elevation in blood pressure. DGL supports the body's natural processes for maintaining the mucosal lining of the stomach and duodenum.

6. Marshmallow Root- is a multipurpose supplement that can be used for respiratory or digestive relief. Like slippery elm, it contains a high mucilage content. It eases the inflammation in the stomach lining, heals ulcers, and treats both diarrhea and constipation by creating a protective lining on the digestive tract. **Dosage**: 300 mg 2 or 3x' a day

7. Caprylic Acid- also known as octanoic acid, is a naturally occurring fatty acid that comes from coconut oil. Calcium and magnesium caprylates act as buffers and may also help slow the dispersion and release of caprylic acid to support its activity throughout the gastrointestinal tract. Caprylic acid is known for its antiviral and antifungal activity. For those who feel that you may be suffering from Candida or yeast overgrowth this is a safe, effective and natural way to treat Candida. **Dosage**: 3600 mg 2x's a day

8. TURMERIC "THIS IS MOST IMPORTANT!" 4000 MG 3X'S A DAY

Turmeric is one of the most effective inflammation fighting supplement known. It accesses 84 inflammatory pathways. Nothing in Allopathic medicine can make that claim.

How long it will take to heal a leaky gut? That, of course, varies from person to person and depends on how the gut became leaky in the first place. Typically, I find that when one follows this program, it should be about a three-month process to achieve total healing.

9. Collagen- may be helpful in assisting sealing up smaller leaks in the intestines. **Dosage**: 1 scoop of powder in juice or a smoothie 2-3x's a day

Note: In cases where open fistulas or large un-healing wounds are in the colon, treatments with the D-Oxygenator have proven successful in 100% of the cases.

DEPRESSION

A total system detox if the first step for relieving and eradicating this conditions.

It is often linked with irritable bowel syndrome. Removal of toxins can and often totally remove all symptoms. (Gut feelings) See also: "Anxiety" protocol.

Then supplement with:
5-HTP 50mg 3 x's per day or 150mg before bed
SAM-E- 200-800mg 2 x's per day on an empty stomach
L-Tryptophan (for depression) 3 caps 3x's a day for the first day. Then, 1-3'xs a day as needed.

L-Theanine (for anxiety) 3 caps 3x's a day for the first day. Then, 1-3 x's a day as needed.

IMMUNE STRENGTHENING

The immune system has many functions. One of its primary functions is to keep the body healthy, by fighting off pathogens that may make us sick. However, another main function of the immune system is to clean house. When your body is rid of toxic debris, there will be little work for the immune system to do.

Another important thing to know: When you are digesting food, your immune system turns off. All the excess energy in the body is dedicated to the digestive system in order to provide the necessary nutrients needed to run and repair the body.

RULE #1: Disease only starts when the body loses its ability to make healthy cells <u>that work.</u>

SUPPLEMENTS FOR THE IMMUNE SYSTEM:

L-Lysine- an amino acid, known as the building block of protein. It is a strong immune system builder. In liquid form, it is absorbed much more readily and completely. Under stress 1000 mg 3-4x's day

Vitamin C- another essential nutrient for the immune. It works synergistically with Lysine.

Lipo-Spheric Vitamin C is the most effective.
Dosage: 5,000-10,000 mg daily. Double, if under duress.

Immune System Mushrooms- a combination of immune supporting mushrooms. The Rishi Mushrooms in the mix rebuild RBCs.

Cordyceps- another mushroom mixture, supports immune, adrenals and prevents kidney stones. These are usually incorporated in the Immune Mushroom mixture.
   Strange thing about Cordyceps: They are actually a spore that infects insects, renders the insect helpless, then grows a projectile out the head of the insect and releases more spores to reproduce itself and spread.

Intra-Max- Liquid vit./min. supplement. 415 nutrients. Essential for providing the building blocks for "healthy cells that work."

Brazilian Mushrooms- (Acarigus Blazai) will triple your NK (natural killer) cells in 48 hours.

Liquid Chlorophyll- Blood builder, oxygenator and blood cleanser.

Iodine- Protects the thyroid gland, is crucial for the brain, needed for producing stomach acid and the best part: it is anti-microbic and a bactericide. If you have enough iodine and a flu virus enters your nostrils, it will be dead before it can get any farther.

Omni-Immune- Kills all pathogens. Boosts and strengthens immune system. 6 drops a day pH's and Voltage- these terms are inner-changeable. The cells must have a constant 7.35 pH-7.45 pH to function properly. This is also saying: -20 mV to -25 mV. This is the voltage needed. The cells must have -50 mV of voltage or (7.66 pH) to reproduce.

Note: When a cell has become acidic, it has <u>lost</u> electrons or voltage. Electrons <u>are</u> voltage.
When a cell has become alkaline, it has <u>gained</u> electrons or voltage.
Note: A *higher voltage* area will always flows to an area of low *voltage.*   (Kirchoff's Law of Conservation.)

GETTING VOLTAGE TO THE CELLS

1. Eat Alkaline foods- vegetables, fruits and other LIVE foods, sprouts, cultured vegetables.
2. Drink Alkaline water- (7.4 pH or above) using an alkaline water machine or Baking Soda.
3. Exercise- muscles moving against one another causes friction. Your cells are electron
generators. When they move, they produce electricity.
4. Petting an animal- electron donors
5. Hugging a tree- electron donors
6. Hugging a person- the electrons will be transferred from the stronger to the weaker area.
7. Walking in the grass barefoot- Earth is a powerful electron donor. No one's voltage area could exceed the Earth's voltage.
8. Moving water- electron donor. Showers stimulate.(electron donor) Baths wear you out.(stealer)

LEAKY GUT REPAIR

1. Have you ever taken an antibiotic at any time in your life?
2 Have you ever used Splenda, even once?
3 Have you, or do you, consume commercially raised meats, beef, chicken, pork and dairy products?
4 Do you experience Stress on a regular basis?
5 Are you overweight and can't lose weight?

6 Do you experience overwhelming cravings for foods that do not support a healthy weight and can't understand why?

7 Do you eat grains like wheat, corn, and rice?

Antibiotics

If you answered "YES" to taking an antibiotic before, you may be surprised to learn just a single round of strong antibiotics can destroy 100% of all the beneficial/friendly "good" bacteria in the Intestinal Tract (aka the GUT)!

These beneficial/friendly bacteria are essential to your health. We are alive and prosper because of the actions of these "good bacteria". Without them - our health suffers.

Here's some things you may not already know:

- Beneficial/friendly "good" bacteria make up nearly 80% of our immune system!
- They also help us digest food for energy and they manufacture vitamins and other substances that support our health and wellness.
- They help with mood management and so many other important functions.

In fact, it can take up to 2 years for these beneficial/friendly bacteria to re-populate and the microbiome to start to function more normally after a round of strong antibiotics – this is especially true when considering the return of the diversity and balance of organisms.

But keep in mind, the health of our beneficial "good" bacteria is only a part of the whole story.

USE OF SPLENDA AND ARTIFICIAL SWEETENERS

If you answered "YES" to ever using Splenda, you may also be surprised that just one packet of Splenda – yes the artificial sweetener that many people think is the "safe one" -can destroy up to 50% of the beneficial/friendly bacteria in the GUT!

If you are trying to cut down on sugar – an excellent idea for GI Health too – using substitutes like Splenda, Aspartame (Equal), etc. are not a healthy alternative. Try using Stevia instead. You may need to shop the brands to find the one you like, but it is well worth the effort!

ANTIBIOTIC USE - Part Two
Many people think, "I haven't had an antibiotic for years, so I am OK." Right? Well…

If you eat commercially raised meats like beef, chicken, pork and use dairy products, you are getting a continuous dose of antibiotics every time you eat these foods.

In fact, 80% of all antibiotics manufactured in the US go into commercially raised meats and dairy.

This means that these beneficial/friendly "good" bacteria are continually exposed to antibiotics! They never stand a chance to maintain levels that are required to support a strong immune system and maintain good health.

Interestingly, Natural casings to make sausage are derived from the GI tract of livestock. The GI Tracts of US livestock can often lack integrity because our cattle (like many of us) suffer from "Leaky gut". These can't be used to make casings. Often casings have to be imported primarily from Argentina or New Zealand where cattle are more organically raised and antibiotics are not used.

CHRONIC STRESS
Stress, especially chronic stress, <u>increases intestinal permeability and GI dysfunction</u>. Most of us live in a constant state of stress and it is such the norm that we don't even realize it or notice it as much anymore.

Stress turns off normal digestive functions (part of the parasympathetic system) because the body's resources are hard-wired to support and turn-on "stress-state" activities (sympathetic system) that enable the body to meet the real or perceived dangers in the fight-or-flight stress response. These include an increased heart rate and blood pressure leading to increased blood flow to the skeletal muscles to support running. The GI muscles relax, and digestive enzymes as well as stomach acid aren't produced.

This fight-or-flight stress worked well for our caveman ancestors who had periodic moments of running for their lives from a Saber Tooth Tiger. They needed all the resources the body could muster for survival and avoid becoming a meal rather than trying to digest last night's meal.

OBESITY AND OVERWHELMING FOOD CRAVINGS
Anything that tips the balance of our Microbiome to favor "bad bacteria" will result in unhealthy food cravings (sweets, starches, carbohydrates) which can eventually lead to obesity.

IMPORTANT CONCEPT – "BAD" BACTERIA THRIVE ON SUGAR, CARBS, STARCHES, AND FATS. However, "Good" Bacteria Thrive on Vegetables, Fruit, and Fiber.

Did you know "Bad bacteria" send messages to our brain to eat foods they crave which are starchy, sugary, fatty foods that promote their health, not ours? If you experience overwhelming food cravings for sweets, breads, pasta, and fried foods– this could be why. Your Microbiome is out-of-balance where "bad" bacteria are in charge.

Stress and Antibiotic exposure tip the balance to favor "Bad Bacteria" too.

Shifting the Balance favoring Good Bacteria can Help Us Maintain a Healthy Weight. Good Bacteria turn off these messages that compel us to eat more food, especially the type of food that makes us gain weight and lead to obesity.

Many people find it easier to manage their weight by eating more foods high in fiber or take a high-quality fiber supplement. Our bodies can't digest the fiber, but the "good" bacteria can – it is their primary food – and when the fiber is in abundance, their colonies thrive.

Eating Grains – Corn, Wheat and other GMO crops are laced with Round-Up.

If you are like most people, you probably eat breads and corn or consume foods that contain wheat or corn. If you eat processed foods at all, this likely applies to you.

Did you know that when you eat commercially grown grains like wheat and corn you are also likely getting a steady dose of "Round-Up"?

That's right, the same chemical you can buy at Home Depot or Lowes to kill weeds.

You probably have never imagined drinking "Round-Up" have you?

Glyphosate – the active ingredient in "Round-Up" - is the choice weed control used in the farming of wheat and corn, along with other grains and GMO crops.

GMO crops have been modified to withstand treatment with Round-Up, so only the weeds die and not the crop plant.

Bacteria (Our Microbiome) and Round-Up

But, Bacteria also die because – like plants - they too are affected by Round-Up.

Americans are now getting a steady dose of Round-Up when they consume these crop foods. These residues also affect the beneficial/friendly "good" bacteria that are supposed to flourish in our GI tracts and keep us flourishing too. Our bacteria, that comprise our Microbiome, are sensitive to Round-Up just like normal (non-GMO) plants.

Intestinal Integrity and Round-Up

Exposure to Glyphosate not only kills the bacteria in our GI Tract, it also promotes "Leaky Gut" because it weakens the tight junctions that hold the cells in our GI tract together.

SUPPLEMENTATION FOR REPAIRING LEAKY GUT

1. L-Glutamine- is an amino acid that is fundamental to the well-being of the digestive and immune systems. Glutamine is great for repairing damage to the gut, helping the gut lining to regrow and repair, undoing the damage caused by leaky gut, and reducing sugar cravings. I recommend 3-5 grams a day.

2. Digestive Enzymes- Digestive enzymes are plant or microbial-based supplements that support the breakdown, absorption, and utilization of macronutrients. Taken with meals, they work with the body's own reduced supply of enzymes to achieve maximum digestion and support intestinal repair mechanisms.

3. Betaine Hydrochloric Acid (HCL)- promotes optimal gastric acidity for support of protein digestion and absorption of minerals and other nutrients such as vitamin B12. There is simple at home test you can do to see if you have low stomach acid and are in need of HCL replacement. Begin to eat a meal and ⅓ of the way into your meal take 650 mg of HCL and then finish your meal. If you experience heartburn, you have sufficient levels of HCL. If you do not experience any burning sensation in your upper abdomen, then you likely would benefit from HCL at each meal.

4. Slippery Elm- It might have kind of a strange name, but slippery elm has been used as an effective gut healer for centuries in the United States. This supplement both contains mucilage and stimulates nerve endings in the body's intestinal tract to increase natural mucus secretion, which is an instrumental part of the stomach's protective lining and helps combat ulcers and excessive acidity in the digestive system. It also contains important antioxidants that help relieve inflammatory bowel symptoms.

5. Deglycyrrhizinated Licorice (DGL)- DGL is an herb that has been used for over 3,000 years in the treatment of digestive issues including ulcers and indigestion. It's made from whole licorice,

but the manufacturing process includes the removal of glycyrrhizin, which can cause an elevation in blood pressure. DGL supports the body's natural processes for maintaining the mucosal lining of the stomach and duodenum.
Dosage: 300 mg 2 x's day

6. Marshmallow Root- Marshmallow root is a multipurpose supplement that can be used for respiratory or digestive relief. Like slippery elm, it contains a high mucilage content. It eases the inflammation in the stomach lining, heals ulcers, and treats both diarrhea and constipation by creating a protective lining on the digestive tract.
Dosage: 300 mg 2 x's a day

7. Caprylic Acid- also known as octanoic acid, is a naturally occurring fatty acid that comes from coconut oil. Calcium and magnesium caprylates act as buffers and may also help slow the dispersion and release of caprylic acid to support its activity throughout the gastrointestinal tract. Caprylic acid is known for its antiviral and antifungal activity. For those who feel that you may be suffering from Candida or yeast overgrowth this is a safe, effective and natural way to treat Candida.
Dosage: 100 mg 2 x's a day

8. Collagen Powder- I scoop in juice or a smoothie can assist sealing up leaks in the gut.
Dosage: 1 scoop 2 or 3 x's a day

9. **Aloe Vera**- Known for its healing properties in ulcers. Very soothing and healing properties.
Dosage: ¼ cup 2 x's a day or 50 mg capsules or powder 2 x's day

The Leaky Gut Diet and 5 Healing Foods

> **#1 Bone Broth** – broth contains collagen and the amino acids proline and glycine that can help heal your damaged cell walls. I've had many of my patients do a bone broth fast for three days to help heal leaky gut and cure autoimmune disease.

#2 Raw Cultured Dairy – contains both probiotics and SCFA's that can help heal the gut. Pastured **kefir**, yogurt, amazia, butter and raw cheese are some of the best.

#3 Fermented Vegetables – contain organic acids that balance intestinal pH and probiotics to support the gut. Sauerkraut, kimchi and kvass are excellent sources.

#4 Coconut Products – all **coconut** products are especially good for your gut. The MCFA's in coconut are easier to digest than other fats so they work well for leaky gut. Also, coconut kefir contains probiotics that support your digestive system.

#5 Sprouted Seeds – chia seeds, flaxseeds and **hemp seeds** that have been sprouted are great sources of fiber that can help support the growth of beneficial bacteria. But if you have severe leaky gut, you may need to start out getting your fiber from steamed vegetables and fruit.

Also, consuming foods that have omega-3 fats are beneficial — **anti-inflammatory foods** like grass-fed beef, lamb and wild-caught fish like salmon.

How long it will take to heal a leaky gut? That of course varies from person to person and depends on how the gut became leaky in the first place. Typically, I find that when one follows the for healing a leaky gut and adds in the above supplements, it should be about a one to three-month process. Intestinal lining cells replenish every 10 days

---

RAISING LOW BLOOD PLATLET COUNT

Platelets are the blood cells that help your blood to clot.

Symptoms may include: Fatigue, easy bruising, bleeding gums,

Easy to obtain supplements for raising platelet count:
B-12- 5000 mcg 1 or 2x's day
Folate- (B9) 1,000 mcg to 2000 mcg daily
Iron- 325 mg 2-3x's a day
Vitamin C- 5,000-10,000 mg 1 or 2x's a day
Liquid Chlorophyll- 1 TBS 2x's day
Note: Folic Acid is a synthetic form of Folate (B9)

Foods that assist in <u>increasing</u> platelets
Mangoes, Green and Red Peppers
Pineapple, Tomatoes
Broccoli, Cauliflower
High in Folate: green leafy vegetables, citrus fruits, legumes, whole grains.

Foods that may <u>decrease</u> platelet count
alcohol
cow's milk
cranberry juice
Tahini

Harder to obtain herbs but VERY effective.
Giloy Herbal Remedy to Increase Low Platelet Count
Ayurveda also talks about another herb, Giloy, which miraculously increases the platelet count. Giloy (Tinospora Cordifolia), also known as Amrita has antibacterial, anti-inflammatory, anti-rheumatic, and anti-allergic actions. It strengthens the immune system effectively. This herb is said to increase the killing ability of macrophages in the body that are responsible for combating micro-organisms and foreign bodies. The stem of giloy plant is used to extract the juice that helps in increasing the count of platelets in the body.

How to make giloy juice to increase platelet count

Get this:

- Giloy stems (4-5 cm long)- 4-5
- Tulsi (holy basil)- 4-5
- Water- 2-3 glass

Do this:

- Soak the giloy stems in water overnight.
- Boil these soaked stems and tulsi leaves in about 2-3 glasses of water till the time the quantity remains half of its original quantity.
- Let it cool down.
- Have it 2-3 times a day

Wheatgrass to Increase Low Platelet Count

Benefits of wheatgrass are no more a secret. Rich in chlorophyll, minerals like magnesium, selenium, zinc, chromium, and antioxidants like beta-carotene, vitamin E, C, B12, as well as iron, folic acid, pyridoxine and various other minerals, amino acids and enzymes, wheatgrass has been accepted as one of the super herbs of our times. It has excellent nutritious and medicinal value along with having anti-anemic properties. All this make wheatgrass juice one of the best remedies for low platelet count. In 2011, a study conducted by the International Journal of Universal Pharmacy and Life Sciences

---

PARKINSON'S AND NEUROLOGICAL TREMORS

Parkinson's Disease occurs when cells in the area of the brain called the "substantia nigra" begin to malfunction and die. These are the cells that produce a chemical messenger called dopamine, which sends information between nerve cells in the brain to produce smooth, coordinated movement.

We have seen remarkable improvement with patients bed-ridden or severely disabled with Parkinson's, my father being one such person. He was unable to get out of a chair or walk without the aid of the wall or stable object to grab or lean against. After the following treatment, he was able to function quite normally. Strangely enough, he quite the supplement treatments and returned from whence he came. I could never figure that one out.

PHASE 1. CLEANSING
Liver/Gallbladder Flush
Intestinal Cleanse
Kidney, Joint, Lymph and Tissue Cleanse

PHASE 2. EATING
Eat small meals and more frequently
Eat mostly raw vegetables and fruits for 1-3 months
After this time period, add fish 3 x's per week
Avoid:
    beef and pork
    ALL fried foods
    Processed foods
    Food additives
    Fluoridated water and products containing fluoride (including
    meds)
    Aluminum cookware
    Deodorant with aluminum
    Shellfish (contain heavy metals)
    Remove ALL metal fillings from teeth (leeches Mercury into
    the bloodstream)
PHASE 3. SUPPLEMENTATION
Lipo-Sheric Glutathione 1 packet (or dose) 3x's day for 3 days
then,
1 packet (or dose) a day until improvement)
Lipo-Sheric Vitamin C- 2 packets (or doses) 3x's day then,
1 packet (or dose) per day
Vitamin E- (400 i.u.) 3x's a day (with meals)
Thiamine- 2,000 mg 3x's a day
L-Tyrosine- 1,000 mg (in the morning on empty stomach)
CoQ10- 400-800 mg daily
Protein Powder- 40-60 grams per day
DHEA- 25 mg per day
Zinc- 50 mg per day (Do not exceed 100 mg per day)
Gingko Biloba- 100 mg 3x's day
Vitamin B-12- 100 mcg in a B-Complex form
NADH (spray) if available) 20 mg a day (energy for the brain)
NADH converts tyrosine into dopamine, which diminishes with
Parkinson's.

ATP (Adenosine Triphosphate) works in conjunction with
    NADH. Take suggested bottle dosage. If possible, get
    NADH w/ATP already combined.
Phosphatidylserine- Brain Fire. Increases mental clarity and
cognitive skills.
1000 mg 1 a day to start with.
Caution: taken after "noon" may cause insomnia.

Note: Large amounts of supplements can be dropped in a
smoothie for easier ingestion. (caps and all)

PROSTATE ENLARGED- TREATMENT
(Benign Prostatic Hypertrophy)
This is a ninety-day program with the exception of selenium,
which one will continue to take indefinitely. If desired results are
not quite achieved, continue until they are.

Zinc-50 mg day 3x's a day
Flaxseed Oil- 9 grams per day
Vit. A (as Beta-Carotene) 300,000 I.U. Per day
Vitamin C- to bowel tolerance
Alfalfa- as directed on bottle

Amino Acids (glycine, alanine and glutamic Acid) 5 grams each
for 90 days
Hydrogen peroxide- 20 drops in 1 oz Aloe Vera Juice 2 x's a
day
Unsweetened Cranberry Juice- 2 pints per day
Saw Palmetto- as directed on container
Selenium- 25 mcg. 3 x's per day (Double this dose for the first
            week, then continue with said dosage.)
Caprylic Acid- to prevent frequent urination.

Note: Caffeine and fried foods are major contributors to frequent
urination, impotence and prostate complications.

SEIZURES
I have had patients come to me, after the doctors say there is

nothing wrong with you. Many patients hear. "It's all in your mind." After this simple protocol, all seizures stop, completely.

We had a young lady come to us who had been having seizures for 2 years, every three hours like clock-work. Her left eye had turned inward 6 months prior and 23 expert doctors could not eradicate the situation. Three of the top ophthalmologists in the country could not explain the condition of the eye, nor provide a cure. Their only recommendation was sniping the optic nerve, letting her eye float around and wear a patch to cover it up.

After being in our facility for three days, ALL seizures ceased, the eye was restored to normal. Instead of wearing an eye patch and suffering seizures the rest of her life, this nineteen-year-old young lady went on to finish school, got her drivers licensed and I'm proud to say has recently received her Naturopathic doctor degree. The following is the protocol we administered to her and to all our seizure patients.

#1 A complete Full Body Detox is step one.
#2 Remove all foods they may cause allergic reactions especially,
   Aspartame, gluten and processed sugars.
#3 D-Oxygenator treatments 2x's day one hour each treatment.

THYROID

"Hypo" or" Hyper" thyroidism are both caused by an iodine deficiency. Hypothyroidism, is deficient in iodine, while Hyper-thyroidism is burning the iodine up faster than it can be made. In either case, iodine is deficient.

No thyroid glandular supplement will show any significant results until the iodine level is first brought up to optimal.

Iodine- 12.5 mg 3-4x's a day for 1 to 2 months, until levels are sufficient.
Thyroid-S (brand and purchasing info in the book Appendix)
Note: It is quite common to find one's weight normalizes after iodine levels are adjusted.

CHAPTER 9

CANCER CAUSE AND CANCER CURES

Did you know: if a cancer cell is able to be detected by any visual means, such as a microscope, it is six to eight years in development?

That's right. It has had ample opportunity to travel many times through your body, via the blood stream. This means, it is quite likely, residence has been taken up in more than one location. This is why it is so important to treat the entire body, not just one specific location.

According to Allopathic medical standards, by law, if you live 5 years after being treated for cancer by conventional medicines, even if you die from the same cancerous condition one day later, you are considered CURED. Even if you're DEAD! They can claim to have "cured" you. Now, by my understanding, "cured" means the condition no longer exists and the body has been restored back to a "healthy state of homeostasis." In other words, as long as you continue to take care of your body sensibly, the condition will <u>never</u> return.

Bernard Jenson is a gentleman I have admired and respected for many years. He was a smart man and a great healer. Dr. Jenson always said,

"The only thing a doctor can cure, is a ham."

Every single day of your life, you will be killing thirty to sixty million "potential" cancer cells, as long as you make a conscious effort to keep your immune system strong and healthy. This means eating the right foods, avoiding the wrong foods, toxins, immune-suppressing additives and continue proper elimination of the colon.

Eighty percent of ALL cancer begins in the colon. The root of the cause, "improper drainage." This doesn't mean the cancer has to metastasize in the colon. It means the toxic waste left in the colon also enters the blood stream, rides around through the body and may metastasize as a tumor in the brain, cancer in the liver, the lungs or any place in the body it happens to adhere.

Again, the weakest and most environmentally adequate parts of the body are the most vulnerable. Let me give you a better understanding of how cancer lives, grows and operates.

To start with, cancer is not a disease caused by a germ, microbe, bacteria, virus or any other outside pathogen, at least not directly. It is a "condition." It is a condition brought about by improper management and care of the body. It is brought on by overloading the body with toxins from poor dietary habits, improper elimination and catastrophic-acidosis, the condition of pH acid-saturation of the tissues and the final breakdown of the immune system. It is your own, once healthy cells, now traitors.

Acidic conditions and improper drainage of putrefied waste, pave the way for mold, yeast, fungus, opportunistic diseases and conditions to take up residence.

Mold yeast and fungus play a big part in the causation of cancer. Certain foods containing mycotoxins actually fertilize mold, yeast and fungi in the body. Just as a diseased plant is the first that bugs will attack, the mold, yeast and fungus begin to attack the body, as they sense the decaying or dying of body tissue due to over acidification.

Here's a brief summarization of some pertinent similarities all cancers have in common:

1. Cancer is anerobic, meaning the infected cell contains no oxygen. Oxygen KILLS cancer.
2. Cancer secretes a protective "fibrin" protein coating around itself, making it fifteen times thicker than a normal, healthy cell's membrane. Radiation can't touch it.
3. A cancer infected cell is highly acidic and continues to move further in the acid direction as it progresses, devoid of any alkaline minerals. Alkalinity KILLS cancer.
4. Eighty percent of ALL cancer begins in the colon.
5. Cancer is only able to metastasize when the immune system fails.
6. Every person kills thirty to sixty thousand cancer cells daily.
7. Cancer loves sugar. Its only food.

Now, let's go over each one of these facts so you will know; exactly what is meant and just what can be done about it.

(1) Why are cancer cells oxygen deprived? A cancer cell is a cell that has gone out of frequency, beyond the range of control by the body's DNA and has been thrown out of the house. It must now go into survival mode. It must learn to fend for itself. It no longer has the body to rely on for the proper nutrients and controlled, minute amounts of oxygen. It must hide, find food and instinctively protect itself from destructive forces. Too much oxygen will kill a cancer cell.

(2) So, it pushes out the oxygen and secretes a "fibrin" protein Coating around itself so no more oxygen can penetrate,

(3) or any other substance such as the alkaline minerals, calcium, potassium, magnesium and sodium, as these too will ruin the environment of the cancer cell or kill it completely, as cancer cannot thrive in an alkaline environment.

(4) Again, 80% of all cancers start in the colon. No matter if it ends up metastasizing in the brain, pancreas, lungs, liver, stomach, kidneys, you can pretty well be assured it came from your colon.

(5) Putrefactive waste, from improper elimination sweeps into the bloodstream via the intestinal walls. Mold, yeast and fungi are present and just waiting for that perfect opportunistic moment, for the immune system to start going down from toxic overload. More garbage continues to pile up until the body's defense system can no longer cope.

(6) Everyone on this planet removes between 30 and 60 million potential cancer cells daily. Your immune system has scouts called "phagocytes" whore primary job is hunting down and destroying these unwanted cells.

(7) **Did you know**: from one sip of soda, or one bite of pie or doughnut, or one scoop of ice-cream or one bite of candy will stop your phagocytes ability to recognize a cancer cell, for nearly two hours? Just one bite of processed sugar stops the defense system from removing any of the 30 to 60 million daily cancer cells trying to accumulate is your system. For someone who drinks sodas all day or pops candy in their mouth all day long or can't pass up the dessert tray anytime its available, merely needs

to multiply how many continuous days this pattern has continued by 30-60 million times 365 days in a year and they can roughly gauge how many unchecked cancer cells are accumulating.

Let's do the math. If a person, for the next ten years spends each day snacking on candy and/or sipping soda, they be letting go, undetected, 356 (days) x 10 (years) x 30,000,000 (cells). That totals up to 109,500,000,000. That's one hundred nine billion, five hundred million, unchecked, opportunistic cancer cells, being gorged with their favorite food, just waiting for that perfect opportunity, that moment when the system's pH level drops into the acid saturation zone and you have just fertilized those cancer cells like Miracle-Grow on houseplants. When the bottom of that pH level drops out, they will have been fed their declaration of war meal and these cancer cells will come down on you like the Indians on Custer at Little Big Horn!

MODERN MEDICINE APPROACH TO CANCER

In the unfortunate event that we have let our body become too acidic with too much concentrated meat protein, sodas, sugar and acid food and drink, our immune system has run down, and the doctor has just dropped the diagnosed cancer bomb. You have just slipped into a temporary mental coma with flashes of your life passing by. He has informed us we have to take "immediate" action; chemotherapy, possibly radiation or may even a piece or two of your body removed. Then we might have a chance at getting rid of this situation, or at least, of prolonging our life a little longer. No promises though, except for the fact you are more than likely going to start feeling like crap in a very short time as you proceed to have your immune system fried out of your body. And you maybe didn't even really feel like anything was wrong with you, until now!

Let us examine the three basic treatments that "advanced" modern American medicine has to offer.

SURGERY

Many times, the first thing a doctor wants to do is start removing body parts. Now, that wouldn't be such a big deal if you could grow the parts back. But that isn't the case and you only have one of whatever it is they are wanting to take out, with the exception of your lungs and kidneys. You obviously needed the part, or it wouldn't be in there.

I realize that decision is essential, even crucial, even unavoidable in certain situations, but not nearly as many part-removals are needed as performed each year.

Then, there is the "biopsy" that is ordered to determine if the pathologist was right or wrong, which is statistically speaking, a 50/50 chance. This is where many non-life-threatening cancers become life-threatening. When you poke into a can of worms, something is going to come out.

What seems to be the predominately popular post-operative procedure now-a-days, is a round of chemotherapy or radiation. Many times, when asked if either one of these procedures will up the anti of survival, the reply is something to effect of, "No, but we just think it's a good precaution to take, anyway."

Its reported many doctors make over 1.5 million dollars each year, just ordering chemotherapy.

Lets look at that next.

CHEMOTHERAPY

Everyone of us knows someone who had been or is undergoing the gruesome torture of chemotherapy. Many of us have a friend or loved one we have lost due to this choice.

We are also all aware of the fact that chemotherapy burns up your immune system. It is made of highly toxic chemicals that are extremely caustic, acidic and a purely man-made chemical.

Now, presuming that the cancer was stimulated in the first place by two factors: toxins and an acidic constitution, why would you choose the two factors that caused the condition, to try and treat the condition? Why would we want to trash even more so, our already toxic, failing immune system and why do we want to make our acidic constitution, even more acidic than it is already, when being over-acidic is what fertilized the cancer in the first place? And why, on God's green earth, would we want to treat a totally organic body with completely man-made chemical compounds that are absolutely poisonous and useless to the human body, when toxic accumulation was the starting point for the manifestation of this disease? Why would we do this? Why would we "choose" this? To this date, not one single "non-toxic" cancer drug has been approved by the FDA.

Do you know the two main causes of death in cancer patients? Its not cancer. They predominantly die from one of two conditions: pneumonia or starvation. Chemo-cremation of the immune system leaves nothing to fight off a simple common cold. And several rounds of chemotherapy leaves the patient with an inability to even keep down a drink of water, let alone a nutritious meal.

And speaking of nutrition, I've been told time and time again, by former chemo patients (some being doctors and nurses) most chemo treatment rooms are stocked with cookies, candies and pastries. Since sugar is cancer's primary food, why would you want to do that? Then the patients were told to go home and eat all the sugar they wanted to build their strength back up after the treatment.... Duh?

Cancer is prompted by missing nutrients. Does our hair fall out because a chem-concoction has just replenished our body with all the necessary and much needed nutrients? Do you dump oil in water and seriously expect it to mix? Would you deliberately dump weed killer in your drinking water and then voluntarily drink it? You can't dump man-made chemicals in a non-man-made-chemical vessel and expect anything but disaster to happen. Why do they leave the room before administering your treatment? And they try to convince you, it's the best thing they've got? Come on!

That's why 95% of everyone that has had chemotherapy is dead after five years. If you don't believe that statistic, call up the Center of Disease Control (1-800-232-4636) and ask them the statistic of cancer survivors, five years after undergoing chemotherapy. Trust me, you won't be pleased with the answer.

Did you know: When you are diagnosed with cancer, you become worth $300,000.00 to the medical community? Whether you live...or not!

RADIATION

Did you know: that mammograms can only detect dense tissue, not cancer, and that a biopsy must be ordered to determine the results, of which 8 out of 10 biopsies come back negative?

Did you know: that the mortality rate of breast cancer in women over 55 was 20% higher in 1955 than in 1970?

Did you know: recently on The Today's Show, they announced a woman over 65 with breast cancer was more likely to die from chemo-induced heart disease, than the untreated cancer, by 65%? They also added, do not get a mammogram unless absolutely necessary. The side effects from the test far outweighs the risk.

Heck, let's do one more…

Did you know: Every cell in the human body has an affinity for the compounds in raw cannabis, and juiced in its raw form, can cure most any ailment of the human body?

One last subject before we get into the alternative options for dealing with cancer. Let's look at what mainstream medicine has to offer and some very interesting information on their relentless, continual usage of radiation.

If you attack a cancer cell with radiation therapy, statistics show there is a better chance of the cancer spreading than if it had not been used at all. Radiation does not have the ability to shrink cancerous tumors, at least, not by removing or killing the cancer cells themselves.

What is happening in actuality, the protective tumor coating is penetrated by the radiation. The encapsulated, easier to kill healthy cells that make up a large portion of the tumor are destroyed, while many of the harder to destroy cancer cells are left intact and free to escape. Hence, we have a smaller tumor, from removal of the healthy cells creating an escape hatch in the casing around the tumor and our cancer spreads. But when our doctor tells us the tumor is smaller, we are elated! And in essence, what has happened is the tumor shrunk only because of the removal of the healthy, no threat cells, while the cancerous cells still remain, as well as the existing problem. So, what have we accomplished?

Statistics show most microscopically detected malignancies would never turn malignant until hit with radiation.

To research more on this subject, read:
"World Without Cancer," by Edward G. Griffin.

Did you know: the "fibrin" protein coating, secreted around the cancer cell makes its membrane 15 times thicker, meaning 15 times harder to kill than a healthy cell?

Before we leave here, I would like to make it perfectly clear, I am NOT criticizing or "bashing" the medical professionals. I very much respect their values, integrity, knowledge, and capabilities. When we get injured and need repaired, they do some pretty miraculous thing. Sometimes beyond believable.

However, I do feel the medical "profession" as a whole, needs to focus more on the humanitarian subject of "health" rather than that of "wealth," and learn the importance of detoxification and restoring the inner terrain of the body back to a state "unfavorable" to disease.

"Plant with good intent and you will reap,
ten times that which you have sewn"

GOING NATURAL

Let's escape from the perspective television "brain-washing" tactical approach of complicated, mainstream, allopathic medicine and look at it from a conceptual approach of logic and common sense or "come-on" sense.

Did you know: just one hundred years ago, alternative "Nature's Health" was mainstream medicine and Allopathic medicine was the "alternative?"

Here's the alternative, logical approach. See if this does not make sense to you.

Reverting back to the above 1 through 5, I will first, give it to you in a nut-shell, then I will go into greater detail.
Remember 1-5.

First, we detox the body and clean the colon, (#4) Then we alkalize the body(#3) Raise the body's oxygen levels (#1) break down the protein secretions around the cancer cells (#2) and finally, begin enhancing the immune system with nutrients (#5). Of course It's not just as simple as that, but in essence, it is quite simple.

Yes, there are times, when in advanced cases such as stage 3 and especially stage 4 cancer, you need a more powerful modality (s) added to the treatment. You need to bring out the BIG GUNS. I'll share some of those big guns shortly.

If you are going to paint a room in your house, do you not first, remove all the furniture, pull all the nails out of the walls and clean off any grease or grime and sand down any rough areas? Then you can reach all the areas and lay down a nice, perfect coat of paint. Same with healing your body.

Depending on the condition of our patient, we begin whatever the chosen treatment, by first doing a complete "full-body" detoxification. We use our personally designed system that works very effectively for cleaning the liver and entire intestinal tract of 10 and 20-year-old waste, resulting in the removal of most toxins and debris that initiated the condition. This can be purchased from: Castle in the Clouds L.L.C. at:
castlesexton@hotmail.com.

Colonics are another option. However, by comparison, the Full Body Detox system, hands down, is the superior method. But we do suggest an ongoing colonics or colema protocol, if possible.

The cleanse is then followed by several days of juice fasting, all depending on the severity of the patient.
(All information for all products mentioned in this book, is located in the appendix or contact Castle in the Clouds L.L.C. at
castlesexton@hotmail.com .

Now that we have swept all the garbage out of the way, we are ready to start filling in those missing nutritional deficiencies. This is done with freshly made organic vegetable juices and a very "high alkaline," mostly raw, vegetarian diet, consisting of the purest organic fruits and vegetables you can find. Again, these should be mostly raw, but some may be steamed or partially cooked. If the patient is in a weakened condition, the food should be more cooked that raw, making it easier on the digestive system until it is able to perform more adequately.

Especially in advanced cases and more severe cases, one needs to absolutely abstain from meat of any kind, until absolutely certain, you are "cancer-free." In all cases, stay away from grease, SUGAR, hydrogenated oils, preservatives, caffeine, wheat, food coloring, processed and GMO foods.

Sometimes, in the case of Stage IV cancer, extra support modalities must be brought in. Here are some proven modalities that can be used in conjunction with the above described protocols.

1. **Indian Black Salve**- can be used topically for skin cancers as well as internally, by capsule. (Highly recommended)

2. **Graviola**- comes from the deep rainforest jungles of the Amazon. Over twenty laboratories have shown Graviola to be more powerful that Adriamycin, a commonly used chemotherapy. Unlike Adriamycin, which can make you very sick, drop your hair and even cause death in some cases, Graviola does no collateral damage. Laboratories have shown it to selectively hunt down and kill twelve different types of cancer including: breast, prostate, lung, colon and pancreatic cancer. It also has proven to be helpful in boosting the immune system and giving the patient a feeling of well-being.

3. **Intravenous Ozone Injections**- saturate the body with oxygen, and we know what that does to cancer cells. However, you will more than likely have to go outside the country for this one.

4. **Joanna Budwig's Flax-oil/cottage cheese remedy**- is always good to include in any cancer therapy. 1/3 cup cottage cheese mixed with 3 TBS flax-oil, taken daily will help the cancer-infected cells return to normal.

5. **High Proteolytic Enzyme Therapy**- is a must when treating cancer. These enzymes eat away at the fibrin coating of cancer cells, making it easier for oxygen and nutrients to enter these cells. (An absolute must) Works great in conjunction with Castle in the Clouds' "high-oxygen-therapy" generators.

6. **High Oxygen Therapy**- oxygen is cancers worst enemy. One of the most effective systems for this treatment is the D-Oxygenator, by Castle in the Clouds L.L.C. Laboratory proven to out-perform hyperbaric chambers by 5-10 times at effectively delivering high concentrations of atomic oxygen subcutaneously, while relaxing in the privacy of your own home.

7. **Essiac Tea**- is another powerful immune builder and cancer fighter. Rene Caisse (Essiac backwards) was healed of breast cancer by this brew of an old Ojibwa Indian Medicine Woman. She started using it on cancer victims with incredible success. It is a <u>must</u> for any cancer therapy.

Its basic ingredients are: burdock root, sheep sorrel, turkey rhubarb and slippery elm bark. A dosage of four ounces one or two times a day is recommended. I personally know a ninety-two-year young gentleman with over two hundred tumors on his body. Of course, the doctors wanted to start whacking away at the tumors, which would surely have done the ninety-two-year old in. The treatment was refused. After one year on Essiac Tea and nothing else, including dietary changes, the tumors are gone. This tea is also a great liver and pancreas detoxifier/regenerator. This tea also has reversal effect on Type II diabetes. (Highly, recommended)

8. **Modified Citrus Pectin**- encapsulates cancer cells and starving them from up-taking their favorite food, sugar. (Highly recommended)

9. **Agaricus Blazei** (Brazilian Mushrooms)- in a twenty-four-hour period will triple your NK cells, the ones that attack and kill the cancer cells.

10. **Rishi Mushrooms**- extremely effective in raising and

sustaining red blood cell count, even during chemo treatments.
11. **Rife Machine**- is one of the most powerful modalities you can have in your arsenal. Through use of selected electronic frequencies, the pathogens are encountered and exploded. In the case with cancer, Rife technology can actually rehabilitate a cancer-infected cell and help restore it back to health. There are many models of Rife machine available out there. Some more effective than others and some are absolutely ineffective.

There are only two categories of Rife machines: (1) the hand-held or galvanic current type that is actually in contact with the patient's skin and (2) the plasma gas tube type that emits electrical frequencies and ultra-sound harmonics throughout the patient's entire body. This is the type Royal Rife used successfully.   (Highly, highly recommended)

!2. **Color Therapy**- very effective in delivering specific electrical frequencies to the deficient body though the use of various colors. Very helpful as a complimentary modality to be used in conjunction with the primary treatment.

13. **Therapeutic Grade Essential Oils**- are very effective as a supporter of the primary modality.

"An ounce of Clove Oil has the antioxidant capacity of 450 lbs. of carrots, 120 quarts of blueberries, or 48 gallons of beet juice." Writes Dr. Stewart, in Healing Oils of the Bible.

Therapeutic-grade essential oils have life. There are inert ingredients called "terpenes" found in essential oils, Monoterpenes, Sesquiterpenes and Phenylpropanoids. One oil may contain all three terpenes.

Monoterpenes: found in peppermint and frankincense can reprogram miswritten information in your DNA. To cancer patients, this is the way cancer starts. One cell with damaged DNA produces another and another and so on.

Sesquiterpenes: are the group that really gives cancer a boot to the behind. They deliver oxygen to the tissues and erase the misinformation of the DNA.

Phenylpropanoids: create unfriendly conditions for bacteria, fungi and viruses. However, their most important function is cleaning the receptor-sites on our cells so that our cells can communicate.

14. **Cesium Chloride**- the BIG GUNS, though seldom heard of, is one of the most powerful and effective alternative cancer treatments available.

Dr. Eric Sartori, of whom I had the privilege and great pleasure of working with many years back, helped refine the cesium protocol to what it has become today. He is a genius-of-a-man and has healed many persons of many cancers using cesium chloride and many others with his extravagant usage of ozone.

Unfortunately, for curing so many persons of life-threatening diseases, he is re-payed by sitting in prison.

Cesium Chloride is a "high alkaline" therapy. Very capable of raising cancer cell's pH upwards of 8.5 pH in 24 to 48 hours. Proven to be 80 to 90% affective on ALL types and stages of cancer.

In conjunction to the liquid cesium/rubidium concoction, one must follow up with a 2:1 ratio of cesium to liquid potassium, (known as Super Potassium) This is used in conjunction with the proteolytic enzyme protocol mentioned earlier, a high alkaline diet, and starting off with a thorough body detoxification regime.

Cesium Chloride/high pH therapy ranks at the top of the list.

Remember, President Ronald Reagan, who was diagnosed with prostate cancer and shortly thereafter, was reported cancer-free? Cesium Chloride.

Cesium Chloride is very frowned upon by the allopathic community. It is very hard to find anything informative (or positive) about it, especially on Google.

It does have its drawbacks. It can be dangerous if used incorrectly. But when used as directed, it can prove to be very effective indeed.

* For more information on Cesium Chloride, go to: www.killcancercells.com or www.thecancertutor.com

The following protocol must researched and used only under the supervision of an experienced practitioner. This is not a suggestion to stop seeing your medical doctor. This information is being supplied for additional possibilities to aid in your search for making the right decision in your fight against cancer. Its your choice!

We have seen many stage IV cancer patients that have been given less than 2-6 months get doctors reports of "cancer-free.'

CESIUM CHLORIDE SAMPLE CANCER PROTOCOL
(Overview)

COMPLETE BODY DETOXIFICATION – 9 to 16 days
LIVER/GALLBLADDER- 1 day
INTESTINAL- 5 days
TISSUE/ KIDNEYS- 3 to <u>10 days</u> (optimal)
BLOOD- (during the detoxing) or do for 2 weeks after beginning eating again)

HIGH ALKALINE DIET 80/20

    AVOID ALL ANIMAL MEATS (including fish and eggs)
    AVOID ALL DAIRY (Except organic yogurt and kefir)
    AVOID ALL **PROCESSED SUGAR**
    AVOID ALL CAFFEINE
    AVOID ALL FOOD COLORINGS
    AVOID ALL PRESERVATIVES
    AVOID ALL GMO FOODS
    AVOID ALL FRIED FOODS
    AVOID CIGARETTES/ALCOHOL

JUICING
3-5 Glasses of fresh vegetable juices daily.

SUPPLEMENTATION
Cesium Chloride/Super Potassium (Essence of Life.com)
800-760-4947 (Start with: 2 Super Potassium and 2 Cesium.)
Liquid Ionic Calcium Chloride-100mg 3x's day
(Amazon/Vita-Cost)
Liquid Magnesium Chloride- 100-200mg 3x's day
(Amazon/Vita-Cost)

Lipo-Spheric Vit. C- (5,000 to 10,000mg day) (Amazon/Vita-Cost)
Selenium- 400mcg per day (Amazon/Vita-Cost)
Zinc- 100mg 2 or 3x's day (Amazon/Vita-Cost)
Milk Thistle- 1 capsule 3x's day (Amazon/Vita-Cost)
D-3- 5,000 I.U. A day (Amazon/Vita-Cost)
Essiac Tea -1/2 C. 3x's day (Make your own)
Graviola- 3 caps 3x's day (Amazon/Vita-Cost)
Black Salve- 1 "00" capsule full at night (Castle Health Retreat)
Omni-Immune- 15 drops 1 or 2x's a day (Castle Health Retreat)
Modified Citrus Pectin- 1 scoop 2x's day (Amazon/Vita-Cost)
Intra-Max Vitamins- ½ cap, 2x's a day (Castle Heath Retreat)
Vital-Zymes- 3-6, 3 x's a day (450 count) (Amazon)
Liquid L-Lysine- 2-3 drops 3x's day(Immune Sys.) (Amazon/Vita-Cost)
Immune System Mushrooms- 3-3x's day (Amazon/Vita-Cost)
Liquid Chlorophyll- 1 TBS 2x's day (Peppermint) (Amazon/Vita-Cost)
Intra-Max-(Liquid Multi-Vit/Min complex) 415 nutrients (Castle Health Retreat)

SUPPLEMENTATION OVERVIEW
INTRA-MAX (Liquid Multi Vit./Min 415 nutrients)
LIQUID CHLOROPHYLL -(Blood cleanser/oxygenator)VIT D3 - (Speeds maturing of cancer cells.) (Can't reproduce)
LIQUID LYSINE- 2-3 drops(Immune System support)
IMMUNE SYSTEM MUSHROOMS- (Strengthens Immune System)
VIT. C- LIPOSOMAL (preferably) as directed (Fights cancer, supports immune)
MILK THISTLE- 2 CAPS (Liver Support)

MODIFIED FRUIT PECTIN- (prevents cancer from up-taking glucose)
BLACK SALVE INTERNAL- 1 capsule per day (min. 45 days) (Kills cancer cells)
OMNI-IMMUNE-15 drops 1 or 2 x's a day (following directions thoroughly) (Kills ALL mold. Yeast. Fungus, viruses, parasites and bacteria in the body) (Supports immune and powerful detoxifier)
(HIGH pH THERAPY CESIUM CHLORIDE-FOR ADVANCED CANCERS (dosages vary)
HIGH OXYGEN THERAPY
   D-OXY BATH- 1 or 2 a day (if checked in) 3 to 5 weekly (if out-patient)
ELECTRONIC MEDICINE
  RIFE MACHINE THERAPY- 1 EVERY 2 or 3 days (2-4-hour frequency sweep)
COFFEE ENEMAS- 1 to 3 per week (LIVER CLEANSE AND SUPPORT)
Note: For weight gain in patients who can't afford to lose any more weight, add 3-5 TBS extra virgin olive oil to smoothies.

There are indeed other effective alternative cancer treatments of varying degrees, High Vitamin C therapy, Mistletoe, Venus Flytrap, Laetrile, raw Cannabis, but listing them all would have us going on page after page. For that reason, I speak only of the ones in which I have worked with and feel most confident in their efficacy.

Regardless of the treatment you choose, you must clean out the body, eat right and think positive. And many of these suggested protocols have proven to be very effective even if one is forgoing conventional cancer treatments such as chemotherapy.

For any "non-medically licensed" practitioners out there working with cancer patients, using alternative therapies, regardless of the modalities you have chosen, you are simply:

"Enhancing the immune system to allow Nature to fend off the cancer and return the body to its natural, healthy state of homeostasis."

Never treat cancer directly.

In dealing with cancer or any life-threatening illness, the immune system is compromised. Whatever the chosen treatment may be, the key is:

"You must keep the healthy cells healthy, to buy time until the immune system can be restored back to a state of self-sustainability."

CHAPTER 10

ARE YOU READY TO ACCEPY A HEALING?

Silly as this question may seem, you'd be surprised at the number of people who are not willing to or are not quite ready to let go of their illness. "Its mine and I want to keep it." Maybe it's a sympathy tool or an attention getter. Maybe it keeps the person from having to work. Maybe they don't think they deserve to be well. Or maybe they just don't believe it <u>can</u> work. Now, there's the real tragedy. Believing is 80% of any protocol. When you believe it, you'll see it! And that's the way the Universe works. That's the way it is set up.

Energy follows intent, or as Albert Einstein put it,

"Nothing can happen until something moves."

Until you put forth the thought, the belief, the intent, nothing is going to happen. And it works from both sides of the fence. If you make statements like, "Well, I'd like it to work, but it probably won't." Guess what? It won't. And do you know why it won't work? Because, "energy follows intent" and "but it probably won't " just set that intent into motion. Its moving alright, but in a negative direction. You're right, it probably won't and all because you made that decision. You just sealed the fate of that intent into doom. And the sad part about it is: you had the same choice with the same chance of success to go the other way, but you chose the negative. Why? Ask yourself, "Do I really want to get well?" See how you answer. And if you decide you do want to get well, keep on reading and as Captain Jean Luc Picard would say, "Make it so!"

HOW TO GET WELL

1. Detox the body through the cleansing of the liver, gallbladder, bowel, blood, kidneys and tissues. Toxins are the cause of 80% of the diseases and ailments you will ever acquire as a human being. Rid your body of the toxins and you will relieve yourself of most any and all ailments, unless viral-

induced. (and we have stuff for that) Toxins interfere with neuro-pathways and energy meridians that can block energy from reaching an organ or system. They can also effect neuro-transmissions, hindering or disabling a message from the brain to reach its intended destination. This can lead to symptoms of cloudy-brain and forgetfulness to petite and Grand Mal seizures.

2.   Replenish the body with the proper natural, organic substances and nutrients needed for rebuilding the body and replacing the missing mineral deficiencies. The body cannot repair itself without the proper building blocks. They must be organic and in their original form as Nature intended for them to be used. Drink plenty of fresh vegetable juices. These will not only alkalize the body, but it's a quick way to wolf down a salad and have almost instant absorption and utilization of its nutrients.

Before putting anything in your mouth, decide if it is nutritionally beneficial or if it will hinder your healing progress. If you don't know, listen to your body. It will signal you through a twitch, a tingle, a cramp or a jaw rush. Don't ignore its signal or it may never signal again.

3.   Drink plenty of water. Every cell in your body needs water to survive. How much water should you drink? Divide your body weight by two and call the answer ounces. This is a ballpark figure of how many ounces of water you should drink on a daily basis. This is a ballpark figure for your daily consumption. Of course, this will vary according to activity and each person's needs. An active person exerting themselves may need twice this amount.

Never get thirsty. This means you have waited too long and have past the point of dehydration.

Add lemon juice to your water whenever possible. This not only helps purify the tissue but is very alkalizing as well. If you can't lay in a bathtub for thirty minutes without shriveling, you are dehydrated. Drink more water.

4.   Get plenty of rest. Your body needs this time to repair itself.

5.   Eat high-electricity or energy-producing foods. You do not

live off the food you eat. You live off the electricity produced by the digestion of that food.

6.   Alkalize your body and keep it that way. A fast way to help with this is to place ¼ tsp of Baking Soda in 4-6 oz of fruit juice. This not only will raise your body's pH level, but it will also aid in the eradication of a virus or bacteria.
Remember: "Germs cannot live in an alkaline environment."

Did you know: Alka-Seltzer is no more than Baking Soda with aspirin and a little Potassium Bromide to give it that theatrical Hollywood fizz? It alkalizes the germs.

7.   Stay at peace with yourself. Be calm. Perform deep breathing exercises. Our cells need lots of oxygen. Meditate at least ten minutes each day. Stress can be very detrimental to the body's healing process.

8. If your digestive system feels disruptive, it is best to go on a fast for a few days. This shuts down the digestive system, allowing it to clear and re-adjust. It also allows the immune system more energy to use in the healing process. You never see an animal eat when they feel sick.

9.   Do some sort of exercise daily. Walking is good. Rebounding on a small trampoline is better. This moves the lymphatic fluid, as it has no pump like the blood has with the heart.
    If you are bed-ridden, have someone give you a lymph massage by pulling their fingers up and down your body, aiming always toward the heart.
    Have them also move your arms, legs and rotate your head. Don't let your muscles lock up and deteriorate.

10. Get fresh air daily, when possible. Fresh air and sunshine have their own healing qualities. A barefoot walk in the cool, green grass is good for the circulation, very stimulating to the soul and is an "electron donor" as the Earth, being a higher voltage area, donates electrons to you, the lower voltage area. This is "Kirchoff's Law of Conservation."

CHAPTER 11

THE CLEANSES

Why should we cleanse? What's in the colon enters the blood. What's in the blood, enters the liver. What's in the blood that leaves the liver, enters the entire body, all of its organs and all of its tissues. How clean you are, is how well you are.

The human intestine is a thirty-foot-long twisting, turning sewer system. It is often very hard for food to make these turns, ending in years of impacted, putrefied, toxic waste. Not only does this impacted waste spew out toxic putrefactive gases, but the blood visits every part of the body about every three hours, including the intestines. In doing so, the blood picks up a supply of this sewage and on its hourly trips begins depositing these toxins to every organ, gland and system in the body. After continuation of these actions, the body becomes auto-intoxicated on its own fecal matter. The blood is contaminated, the polluted organs begin to fail and before long you are at the doctors wanting to know why suddenly (after twenty or thirty years) you feel like crap. Because you are full of it!

How often do you need to cleanse?

If you only do it ONCE, you have removed most of the accumulated waste over your entire lifetime. You have taken charge of your health and will most likely rid yourself of most ailments and causation of those ailments. Once is a major step in the right direction. However, we recommend once a year, if not every six months to obtain and retain maximum health benefits. Cleansing is not an excuse for continued eating abuse. Eat healthy.

Who will benefit from this cleanse?

Everyone! Complete body cleansing is crucial for chronic illnesses. It is crucial for optimizing the efficacy of any health protocol. Patients have experienced amazing results from many illnesses ailments from weight loss to life-threatening diseases.

Should I stop my medication during the cleanses?

That is a decision <u>you</u> must make. This must be of your own choosing. If you are on medications that are absolutely prolonging your life or are administered to control a life-threatening condition, such as high risk for blood-clot formation, by all means, continue that medication. For high blood pressure, diabetes, cholesterol, etc., here is our suggestion and remember, this is only a suggestion: We suggest, for less serious medications, you restrain from taking and check your BP or sugar level periodically. If it raises to a level of concern, take a half dose. If that is not enough, take the second half. Do this until the medication is no longer needed. Generally, your blood pressure and sugar levels normalize almost immediately. If you feel reluctant, ask your doctor's advice.

What effects should I expect after cleansing?

Approximately 80-90% of every illness or malady one will acquire during a lifetime will be a result of toxins and toxic waste buildup in the body. Cancer, diabetes, high blood pressure, COPD, Autism, Parkinson's, Alzheimer's, weight gain, skin conditions, glandular and hormonal issues, depression and neurological disorders all have an underlying root cause of toxic waste in the body. This is just a small list of the ailments caused from toxins. Fibromyalgia, MS, Lupus and most every other auto-immune disease can be greatly improved and most often eradicated with continued cleansing along with a clean, healthy dietary protocol.

Note: It is crucial that the cleanses be done in order and as laid out. So, please, read the directions carefully and in their entirety before proceeding, as you want you to experience the full benefits, amazing results and optimal health that the many others before you have achieved. It is possible to experience brief discomfort or flu-like symptoms as the body detoxes. It may precipitate going through a healing crisis.

To your health!

#1   <u>**Twenty-Four-Hour Liver/Gallbladder Cleanse**</u>

Your liver is your blood filter. There is one quart of blood in your liver at all times, getting de-putrefied, detoxified, cleansed and rejuvenated. Every toxin, medication and nutrient that passes through your lips, passes through your liver. Having nowhere to really go with all this accumulative crud, except for releasing it back into the body, which it doesn't want to do, it begins to overload. With storage room filling up, it begins to allow some of the new crud to get by and into the bloodstream. This can become very dangerous.

Your liver produces bile, used to break down certain elements, and it sends it to the Gallbladder for storage. From the owner's poor eating habits, the gallbladder will begin to fill up with gallstones. These are cholesterol-coated, partially-processed proteins that can sometimes lodge in the gallbladder. Especially, when the bile duct has been clogged up. First signs of a problem are frequent feeling nauseous after eating.

When we want to regain control over our health, especially when we are very ill and even more so when we are facing a life-threatening illness, we want to first, cleanse our liver and gallbladder. This method is one of the quickest, easiest and most effective method I have found.

The times suggested to perform each step are not crucial and may be adjusted to fit one's schedule. You may want to start earlier or later in the day. However, the spacing between steps IS crucial. Please, follow each step exactly.

24 HOUR LIVER FLUSH/GALLSTONE REMOVAL

Do even if you have no gallbladder! Adjust all the times according to when you start.

DAY 1

6:00 A.M. - Drink 1 Quart distilled water

7:00 A.M. - Drink as much unfiltered APPLE JUICE as desired (2 quarts min.)

(We suggest "Simply Apple" brand or any health food store brand)

12:00 NOON- No more fluids except distilled water

5:00 P.M. – Dissolve 2 TBS Epsom Salts in 1 Quart distilled water, drink (for taste sake: dissolve the salts in 4 oz water' add the juice of ½ lemon and drink. Follow with the remainder of the quart of distilled water.)

9:00 P.M. – In a jar with lid, Mix 4 oz. fresh squeezed lemon juice/4oz. Virgin olive oil
Shake enough to blend. (5 to 10 sec.)
Drink quickly while standing. (This step to be performed just before lying down to sleep.)

- To avoid possible nausea, place ¼ tsp baking soda in ½ C. apple juice or water and drink before oil mixture.

Drink one more of these baking soda mixtures after the oil mixture as well. This will combat the tendency for nausea.

***Lie on right side to sleep and prop pillow behind back as to retain position   (This step is Not crucial)**

***Upon arising, REPEAT: EPSOMS SALT STEP elimination of stones will occur during next bowel movement..**

**To make the Epsom Salts more palatable, place 4-6 oz of the water in a small glass, add the Epsoms and ½ fresh-squeezed lemon juice. Stevia may also be added. Chase with remainder of the quart.*

The liver will receive its energy for cleansing about 3:00 am and the gallbladder around 3:30 am. It is important to keep the oil/lemon juice concoction down until this time. If you are unsuccessful in doing so, it is suggested you repeat this cleanse.

*** For optimal liver function and health, it is advisable to do this cleanse every six months.**

INTESTINAL CLEANSE

The intestines, as we know, are nothing more than a sewer running right down the middle of our body. However, a lot of important stuff goes on in this sewer! Our food is broken down and nutrients are separated and absorbed through the intestinal walls and into the bloodstream. This is how we get our nourishment.

We have some thirty feet of intestines winding around, back and forth inside our body that the food must travel. Some of those turns in there can be rather sharp, and feces can sometimes get caught trying to make one of these turns and not make it all the way to the end of the road, or the colon. It then lies there and begins to putrefy. This in turn lead to putrefied matter beginning to leak toxic gases into our intestines, then through the intestinal walls and on into the bloodstream. Which, in turn, is circulated to every part of your body. We Are now becoming "auto-intoxicated." I know you know this already because I have repeated it several times, but I want to be sure you get it. Get it?

Then we begin to feel tired. More food begins to form on the walls of our intestines and before long, we are unable to pass nutrients through the cemented walls.

Soon, our intestines begin filling up and bowel movements become fewer and fewer. (Which, by the way, you should be having at least three times a day.)

Next, we begin having pains in our midsection that soon become excruciating. The doctor diagnosis us with, "Diverticulitis," pockets protruding in the intestines or even worse, "Colon Cancer."

So, let's clean that sewer out once in a while and be a little more selective in what we eat.

There are a number of ways to clean your colon.

Colonics- are basically a pressure-washing, using low pressure water, pumped into the colon and expelled. A series of these procedures is generally needed. These machines are expensive so, you might want to seek out a colon therapist.

Colemas- are basically the same thing as a colonic, only you do these at home, with generally a 5-gallon bucket of water.

Coffee Enemas- are another way to go, although these are considered more of a liver detox than a colon cleanse. They are basically an enema taken with coffee whereas, you lie on one side for 5 minutes, then the other, then the back and run back to the toilet and expel.

Store-Bought Colon Cleanses- as well as the ones on T.V., we find generally to be ineffective.

At **Castle in the Clouds**, we prefer our own cleanse, which we have worked for many years perfecting. We put it against ten straight colonics on ten persons after ten days of juice fasting and after the ten-day round of colonics, they each did our 5-day colon cleanse and each person had an average of 5 bowel movements a day for each of the 5 days. We consider that pretty effective. We have found them to outperform any other form of cleanses available. They've totally replaced our colonics department.

For ordering information: see the appendix section in the back of this book.

This is the second cleanse.
DAYS: 2-6 (5 days)

INTESTINAL CLEANSE

***The Intestinal Cleanse is to be started two to three hours after the second Epsom Salts dose.**

<u>Directions</u>

1. In a small jar with a lid: add 4-6oz Apple Juice + 1 level Tablespoon of Powder.
Shake well and drink IMMEDIATELY. Will turn to cement in 2 minutes.
2. Follow each of these drinks with 8oz of distilled water. (This prevents backup and blockage.)
3. You will drink one of these drinks every three hours, totaling 5 drinks a day.
4. Each night before bedtime, take 3 digestive stimulants (included in the container.)
5. This is to be continued for 5 days. This will be a total of 25 drinks in the next five days.

During this cleanse, you may have smoothies, fresh veggie juices, herbal teas and the following broth:.

Potassium Broth Recipe:

2 to 4 red potatoes, 2 carrots, 1 bunch parsley

1 medium onion, 2 celery stalks

1-quart distilled water + 1 vegetable bouillon cube

2 TBS Bragg's Amino Acids (optional for flavor)

To prepare:

Coarsely chop all ingredients.

Dissolve vegetable cube in boiling water.

Reduce heat to low and add all ingredients. Cover and simmer 30 minutes.

Strain and drink.

Note: For a quicker version, simply dissolve a vegetarian bouillon cube in boiling water. Add some

Bragg's Amino Acids for flavor. Garlic and or ginger may be added for additional flavor.

LEMON/WATER/MAPLE SYRUP CLEANSE

Better known as "The Master Cleanse," this cleanse is wonderful for detoxifying the body's tissues. Using lemons or limes, both being the only food source on the planet with an opposite ionic spin of all other foods. Toxins are pulled out of the tissues like a magnet and into the kidneys for expulsion.

Raw Maple Syrup contains all the nutrients the body needs in perfect proportion. It also acts as your food source or your carbohydrates.

These ingredients are placed in distilled water, resembling a very fine gourmet lemon-aid. For those who want to speed their metabolism, for aiding in weight-loss, cayenne pepper may be added. At **Castle in the Clouds**, we do not use the cayenne, as we are going strictly for the cleansing effect. We have stronger means of weight loss in our repertoire. However, with or without the cayenne, you <u>will</u> lose weight.

This is the third cleanse!

LAST CLEANSE (DAYS 7-9 minimal results or DAYS 7-16 for maximum results)

MASTER CLEANSE

***This cleanse is to be performed <u>last,</u> after finishing the 5-day Intestinal Cleanse.**

This cleanse will clean up remaining debris, joints, tissues, kidneys, skin, eyes and brain.

If you feel light headed during this cleanse, chew up 5 black grapes and spit out the pulp. Fixes carb drops in seconds.

Ingredients:

1 GALLON Distilled Water

1 Cup FRESH SQUEEZED lemon juice (Cannot use bottled lemon juice on ANY cleanse. MUST BE FRESH.)

½ to 1 Cup Pure Maple Syrup (Spring Tree or Maple Grove brands are our suggestions)

Mixing Instructions:
Remove 2 cups from 1 Gal distilled Water jug and save to the side.
Add the Lemon Juice and Maple Syrup

Dosages:
Drink 8 oz of this mix, every hour, on the hour, for 8 hours. (This is 64 oz. or 1/2 gallon.)

This is to be done daily for a minimum of 3 days.

We suggest for a chronic, severe or stubborn ailment, do the 10 full days of this Master Cleanse for max benefits.

Note: The ½ Cup dose of Maple Syrup is for those who want to lose weight. If you are feeling tired, you may want to add 1 whole cup of the Maple Syrup.

½ gallon (64oz) is the minimum daily dose. There is NO maximum. If you're hungry, DRINK

Note: To prevent possible electrolyte loss, we suggest drinking coconut water several times a day during these cleanses or add an electrolyte supplement.

Note: Keep black grapes on hand during these cleanses and at any time, particularly with the Lemon/Water/Maple Syrup cleanse, if you feel light headed or weak, take 5 of these grapes, chew them up, swallowing the juice and spitting out the meat. This will prevent or stop carb drops.

BLOOD CLEANSER TEA

Here is a wonderful blood cleansing tea I learned from a fantastic herbalist, Rosemary Gladstar.

Many toxins, like those toxic gases seeping from your colon, can enter the bloodstream, circulate throughout one's body and cause various illnesses. They can range from blood disorders, to quite severe illnesses such as lupus and cancer. In order to remove any pre-existing toxins or ones that may have been forced out into the blood and still remain, it is wise to clean the blood after performing the previously mentioned cleanses. You can eat with the Blood Cleanser Tea. Just eat clean!

You can buy the following ingredients in any health store that sells loose herbs, or order on line. Do not try and use tea bags. It will not work.

Ingredients:
2 TBS- Burdock Root
2 TBS- Echinacea Root
2 TBS- Nettle Leaves
2 TBS- Red Clover
2 TBS- Elder Flowers
2 TBS- Peppermint

Preparation:

Bring 6 cups distilled water to a boil.

Add- Burdock and Echinacea, reduce heat. Cover and simmer for ten minutes

Add-Nettle. Cover and simmer ten more minutes

Add- Red Clover, Elders and Peppermint. Cover and simmer ten more minutes.

Remove from heat. Let cool.

Strain through a sieve and into a container.

Keep refrigerated.

Dosage: Drink ½ Cup 3 x's a day for two weeks. Make as needed.

CHAPTER 12
RULES OF EATING

1. Chew your food well. Your saliva is the first stage in the digestion process. The more we masticate and break down our food, the less work there is for our digestive system. This means more energy for our physiological functions.
2. Don't eat unless you are hungry enough to eat nutritional, wholesome foods.
3. Don't overeat when you do eat. This adds much extra work and stress on the digestive system. It is also a sure way to guarantee improper and incomplete food processing. It is also a good way to put on extra pounds.
4. Don't eat too fast. Shoveling food in faster than the brain can register fullness to the body, will lead to rule #3, overeating. Take your time and enjoy the bite you have in your mouth before loading up for the next bite. If need be, set your utensil down between bites.
5. If you feel out of balance in mind or spirit, don't eat. If you don't feel good on the mental level, your digestion will not work properly on the physical.
6. Don't eat if you eat when you are upset, unhappy, tired, sick, depressed, overheated or in pain. Food digestion takes a tremendous amount of energy. When you ingest food under these kinds of conditions, you are robbing the body of much needed healing energy. Rest is more important than eating in these types of situations.
7. Do not eat greasy or fried foods. These foods are full of free-radicals, devoid of nutrients and lecithin, due to the molecular altercation of the heated oils. These foods lead to heart disease and increase the risk of cancer as well as clog the arteries and damage other vessels as well as the digestive tract.
8. Drinking liquids with meals is not the best thing to do, as they dilute the digestive enzymes. If you do drink with meals, cold drinks should first be warmed in the mouth before they are swallowed. The digestion process requires heat to function properly. A cold beverage will quickly lower the body temp.,

Thus hindering the digestive process. It is best to drink a glass of water 30 minutes before eating and 1 ½ hours after.

9. Do not combine animal proteins and other acid-stimulating foods with carbohydrates at the same meal. Proteins need an acidic environment during the first stages of digestion, the stomach. Carbohydrates need total alkalinity throughout the entire process. Introducing protein during the digestive process of a carbohydrate, will instantly halt the carbohydrate digestion. This causes incomplete digestion and instant carb fermentation. This is turn leads to gas, bloating and non-absorption of important nutrients.

10. Eat fruits and vegetables at least thirty minutes apart from each other. Mixing these two food groups at the same time can lead to fermentation, gas and bloating.

11. For optimal health, stay entirely away from those foods containing: preservatives, food colorings, hydrogenated oils, processed sugar, caffeine, MSG, high salt, bleached white four and gluten. (even if you think you have no intolerance)

12. Eat 80% alkaline diet: 6 vegetables/2 fruits/1protein/1 starch. 60% of your diet will be raw. I'll explain the whole thing in the following "80/20 Alkaline Diet" section.

13. If you can't pronounce it, DON'T EAT IT!

14. NEVER microwave! In two seconds the molecular structure of food is altered, rendering it unusable by the human body. In 1 minute, ALL nutrients and enzymes are destroyed and all that is left is a pile of free radicals.

THE 80/20 ALKALINE DIET

This is the perfect diet for any constitution, no matter what your blood-type, no matter what your body-type. Let's not even call it a "diet." Its not a diet, it's a way of life. If you're overweight, you'll lose the weight naturally, stopping when and where Nature decides and keep it off. If you are ill, this will help you heal. Your body will continue to rebuild and repair until is it in the most optimal "disease-resistant" state of health possible.

Rule #4:

"If you maintain an external pH of 7.4 pH, you cannot get sick."

Germs, virus and bacteria cannot live in an alkaline environment. And just how does one go about achieving this wonderful state of blissful well-being? By eating this 80% alkaline/ 20% acidic combination of foods consisting of 6 vegetables, 2 fruits , 1 protein and 1 starch in equal portions, daily. By portion, I mean equal amounts: 6 TBS + 2 TBS + 1 TBS + 1 TBS or 6 cups + 2 cups + 1 cup + 1 cup, etc.

One more way of looking at it would be:

Take your daily food consumption, let's make it round like a pie, cut it into 10 equal slices. 6 of those slices or 60% will be veggies, 2 slices or 20% will be fruits, 1piece or 10% will be protein and the last piece or 10% will be starch. See, we're still getting to eat pie… not really!

By now you're probably thinking, "What the ….? I'll explain.

For the sake of simplicity, let's say ALL vegetables and fruits are _alkaline_ and ALL proteins and starches are _acidic_. There are exceptions to this rule, but for now, let's just keep it simple.

Here is your healthy eating equation for **Rule #4**:

"6 vegetables + 2 fruits, 6 + 2 = 8 or 80% (alkaline)
1 protein + 1 starch, 1 + 1= 2 or 20% (acidic)"
(60% of your vegetables should be raw and 40% cooked)

Remember, we are now talking foods that form alkaline and acidic "ash," not calciums that produce "electro-magnetismic energy," as with the liver and calcium.

"Okay, now you're just talking crazy gibberish!"

Let me explain this one.

"Thanks, I appreciate that, Doc!"

What is acid/alkaline ash? Just as wood-ash residue is left from a fire, so is the food-ash residue from the sugars being burned off of the foods ingested, as your body uses or burns them up.

So, where the "external body," (your skin and tissues) category is concerned, unless you have a tissue biopsy performed, (and no one does that) it must be "ass-u-med" (I know, the "u" between "ass" and "me") by your diet alone, after eating this way for approximately 2 months, your external pH is maintaining around a 7.4 pH value.

There are NO fluid tests at this time, that can actually measure your "tissue" pH. We can test the urine and tell what the urine pH is, test the saliva and even test the blood. But there are no fluid tests that tell you the exact pH of the tissue.

I want to repeat this one more time, because I want you to know how important this is to remember and how absolutely POWERFUL this knowledge is:

"When you retain an external pH of 7.4, you CAN'T get sick." No bug, germ, virus or bacteria will want to take host in your body, because you will make them sick. If you have your children eating in this manner, no more missing school because of colds or the flu. (sorry kids!)

"A penny under the tongue can still spike a fever."

Shhh…don't tell your parents that one! It'll be our secret.

Now, to help you along with this new way of eating for health and wellness, I have included a few food charts to help keep thing straight. In case you are unsure, you can just look it up on the chart. There are also charts on substitutions of ingredients for cooking as well. You'll see how to turn any Betty Crocker recipe into a healthy recipe.

Soon, you will establish certain foods you like and ones you don't. Then you don't need the charts. Then you don't need to keep reading labels.

One last thing before move on:

Eating is fun. It should be fun. Take this 80/20 eating regime and tailor it to your likes and needs. Don't make eating such a hassle, such a pain in the "arse" that you would rather DIE than to eat healthy. Just stay as close as possible and as healthy as possible to the original format.

Here's the eating plan, then the charts. Eat well, live well!

<u>HEALTHY EATING PLAN</u>

(These are merely suggestions to help you get started on course.)

(If you a cancer patient, EXEMPT ALL ANIMAL MEAT, especially stage IV cancer)

Upon Rising:
1. 2 TBS- Liquid Chlorophyll in 6 oz. Grape juice.
2. Take any chosen supplements.

Choose from any of the following:

1. Yogurt w/1 tsp. Each; wheat germ, lecithin granules, sesame seeds and Brewer's Yeast + two kinds of fresh fruit.
2. Whole grain cereal w/almond, rice or soy milk, lecithin granules and fruit.
3. Fruit smoothie w/protein powder, flax oil and lecithin granules.
4. Whole grain pancakes with Raw Maple Syrup, w/yogurt, butter and lecithin.
5. Egg, lightly poached or 3 min. boiled w/whole grain toast or whole wheat muffin.
6. Oatmeal w/pure Maple Syrup. Lecithin granules and an apple.
7. Fresh fruit bowl w/flax seed oil, tahini, lecithin granules, honey. Top w/ yogurt.

Choose from the following:

Mid-morning:
1. Green-Drink (mixture of 3-4 green veggies or Wheatgrass, Barley Green, etc.)
2. Sun Chlorella
3. Potassium Broth
4. Ginseng or Gingko Tea
5. Yogurt w/nuts and or seeds.
6. Miso Soup (Watch the salt) w/snipped sea veggies (opt.)
7. An Apple.

Choose from the following:

Lunch:
1. Fresh green salad (6 veggies) and brown rice
2. Baked or broiled fish w/steamed vegetables
3. Whole grain veggie sandwich
4. Steamed vegetables and brown rice
5. Roast turkey sandwich on whole grain bread
6. Whole grain pasta
7. Vegetable soup w/whole grain muffin

Choose from the following:

Mid-afternoon: Take another group of chosen supplements, plus:

1. Herbal Tea
2. Yogurt w/fruit and or nuts
3. Crunchy raw veggies with Hummus dip, bottled water
4. Fresh fruit with soy or veggie cheese
5. Soup broth
6. Carrot or other fresh vegetable juice
7. Protein smoothie

Choose from the following:

Dinner: Chosen supplements plus:
1. Steamed vegetables w/tofu and brown rice.
2. Vegetable pasta
3. Baked or broiled seafood or fish
4. Light vegetable Quiche w/soy or veggie cheese
5. Vegetarian pizza made with soy or veggie cheese and whole grain crust
6. Oriental stir-fry (using lemon juice instead of oil) brown rice
7. Light sup and brown rice and or Wasa Bread

Choose one:

Before bed:

1. Cup of herb tea, such as Chamomile (relaxing tea)
2. Cup of hot vegetable broth.
*** Combined discipline and diligence with this eating regime will reward you with optimal energy and disease-free health.**

ALL biological life on this planet has the most optimal working energy with a pH of 6.4 pH.

The Urine and Saliva pH governs the efficacy of the liver, digestion and overall health of your inner terrain.

You are an electric being. You should learn the following:

"You do not live off the food you eat. You live off the energy produced by the digestion of that food."
    Learn to eat "electricity-producing" foods. These are foods that are still living with enzymes intact, such as fresh, raw veggies, fruits and sprouts.
    Cooked foods, such as dead animal, have no enzymes to digest the food. Therefore, your body must manufacture digestive enzymes and that takes so much energy, you want to take a nap after eating. Eat live, spark-producing foods. You will build up a never-ending reserve of energy.

DO NOT fall for the misconception that you should get your body as ALKALINE as possible. This will manufacture you many maladies such as Kidney Stones, Upper Respiratory ailments, sinus problems, constipation, cannibalism of the upper portions of your organs, hardening of upper organ tissue and the list goes on and on. Keep your Urine and Saliva pH's respectively at 6.4 pH.

Too acidic causes, nervousness, diarrhea, susceptibility to germs, viral and bacterial infections, wearing out of myelin nerve sheath, cold all the time. The body exterior may be kept at 7.4 pH for disease resistance, but the urine/saliva must remain 6.4 pH. The term "pH" stands for "Potential Hydrogen."

STARCHES, CARBS, FATS AND PROTEINS LIST

<u>STARCHES</u>

Wheat	Irish Potatoes
Buckwheat	Sweet Potatoes
Rye	Banana Squash
Oats	Hubbard Squash
Barley	Pumpkin
Corn	Banana
Rice	Sago
Peanuts	Tapioca
Chestnuts	Dry Peas
Yams	Dry Beans

<u>COMPLEX CARBOHYDRATES</u>

Carbohydrates are composed of sugars, starches and cellulose.

All fresh vegetables: Fresh or frozen, eaten raw or steamed. Green vegetables are

by far the top choice, but all are on the menu. All foods except animal protein contain carbohydrates.

The following gives a percentage of usable sugar energy.

5%	**10%**	**15%**	**20% or more**
Artichokes	Beets	Green Beans	Baked Beans
Asparagus	Carrots	Lima Beans	Bread
Broccoli	Kohlrabi	Parsnips	Brown Rice
Brussels Sprouts	Onions	FRUIT	Green Corn
Cabbage	Pumpkins	Apples	Potatoes
Cauliflower	Squash	Apricots	Shell Beans
Celery	String Beans	Blueberries	Lentils
Cucumber	Turnips	Cherries	Lima
Egg Plant	FRUIT	Currants	Navy
Endive	Blackberries	Huckleberries	Soy
Leeks	Gooseberries	Pears	Shredded Wheat
Lettuce	Lemons	Raspberries	Whole Rye
Mushrooms	Oranges	NUTS	FRUIT
Okra	Peaches	Almonds	Bananas
Radishes	Pineapple	Beechnuts	Plums
Rhubarb	Strawberries	Walnuts (English)	Prunes
Sauerkraut	Watermelon		NUTS
Swiss Chard	NUTS		Chestnuts
Tomatoes	Black Walnuts		Peanuts
Watercress	Brazil Nuts		
FRUIT	Filberts		
Ripe Olives	Hickory		
Grapefruit	Pecans		
NUTS			
Butternuts			
Pignolias			

SIMPLE CARBOHYDRATES

Simple carbohydrates are basically processed sugar with no nutritional value.

Examples: Processed/Refined Sugar Candy Bars Twinkies Little Debbie Cakes, Ice Cream, Store-bought pies and cakes, etc.

<u>FATS</u>

(Exist chiefly in animal products)

Milk
Eggs
Animal Meat
Seeds (good fat)
Nuts (good fat)
Dairy
Avocado (good fat)
Olive Oil (good fat)

<u>PROTEINS</u>

The largest molecule of the biochemical world, proteins are made up of nitrogenous long chains of

"Amino Acids". There are 20 amino acids, 8 of which are "essential", meaning the body doesn't produce them and must be supplemented through dietary intake. The body only absorbs 20-30% of the protein from meat, but 85-95% of the protein from plants, nuts and seeds. Protein foods are divided into two main groups; animal protein and vegetable protein.

Soy Beans	(a complete protein)
Tofu	36% protein
All Beans	25% protein
Legumes	9-28% protein
Alfalfa Seeds	35% protein
Mung Beans	27% protein
Sunflower Seeds	27% protein
Lentils	26% protein
Split Peas	26% protein
White Beans	24% protein
Garbanzos	24% protein
Egg Whites	10.62 – 13.63% protein
Milk	3.3% protein

Yogurt   10% protein
Cheese   16% protein
Beef (lean)   23% protein
Fish   22% protein
Chicken   21% protein
Turkey   23% protein
Hard Wheat   14% protein
Whey Protein Isolate   79% protein
Mock Meat   18-24% protein
Spirulina Algae   55-77% protein

Proteins are categorized into: Antibodies, Enzyme, Messenger, Structural, Transport/Storage..

<u>SUBSTITUTING FOODS</u>

<u>DAIRY PRODUCTS</u>

Milk and Cream:

Soymilk- plain or vanilla; substitute equal amounts for milk or cream. (Buy Non-GMO)
Yogurt and water mixed to the consistency of milk-use in equal amounts for buttermilk.
Kefir (liquid yogurt) may be substituted in equal amounts for milk, buttermilk, half n half.
Almond Milk or other nut milk, an excellent substitutes in gravies, soups, sauces, cereal.
(To make : 1 tsp. Almond Butter, 1 tsp. Honey, 1 Cup water. Blend in blender.)
Tahini Milk- made by adding 1 TBS Tahini to 8 oz water and a little Honey.
Rice Milk- use as equal amounts for milk recipes.
Fruit Juices- use on cereals to replace milk.
Water- in place of milk in hot cereals and recipes for a dry, crunchy taste instead of moist.
Lecithin Granules- mix into sauces or gravies to emulsify and thicken without milk / cream.

Ice Cream:

Rice Dream and Soy-based ice cream substitutes are available.
Soy Milk- simply freeze in bowl, 3-4 hours, or freeze a smoothie
made with Nut Milk.
Lecithin Granules- mix 1-2 TBS into frozen desserts to emulsify
without milk or cream.

Cheeses:

Soy, Rice, and Veggie Cheeses are great non-dairy substitutes.
Veggie melts the best.

Tofu-marinated and sliced for use on sandwiches.

Kefir Cheese- use as substitute for Cream Cheese or Cottage
Cheese.

Yogurt Cheese- place 16oz plain yogurt in cheese cloth and hang
over sink. It takes approx.14-16 hours for the whey to drain and
you have Yogurt Cheese! Save and use the whey in soups and
stews. High nutrition and good!

Note: The "Un-Cheese Cook-book" on Amazon is FULL of non-
dairy cheese recipes.

Sour Cream:

Yogurt (plain)- for a slight added tang, add lemon juice.

Half and half mixture of Yogurt and Mayonnaise

Tofu Mayo Recipe: ½ TBS lemon juice, ½ tsp Dijon Mustard (or
light miso) ½ tsp Sesame

Salt, 2 TBS Olive Oil, 4 TBS plain Yogurt and ½ tsp Tarragon
Vinegar. Use also as sub for Cream Fraiche.

Egg Substitutes:

Egg Replacers- from health food store (most commercial brands, as well as creamers are made from plastic powders.)

Dry yeast or Sourdough- use as leavening agent in place of eggs.

Starchy vegetables, Applesauce, Flaxseed and water mix, or Almond Butter, used as a substitute binding agent for eggs.

Tofu- fresh and crumbled in place of scrambled eggs, and in some recipes.

MEAT

Meat Substitutes:

Soy Turkey
Soy Chicken- found ground, nuggets and sliced
Soy Ground Beef
Soy Pork- sausages, bacon, Canadian Bacon slices, Pepperoni slices
Tempeh- buy pre-seasoned or do it yourself- substitute for red meat.
Falafel- or grain burger mixes; mix with water as directed and sub for any ground meat.

GRAINS

Wheat, Gluten and Yeast Substitutes:

*Yeasted bread substitutes: Rye, rice cakes, Mochi, Corn Tortillas, Chapatis, Essene Bread

Flat Breads, Quick Breads and Pancakes made with Baking Powder.

* Wheat Pasta Substitute- Corn, vegetable pasta, 100% Buckwheat Soba Noodles, frozen
then thawed Tofu. Freezing Tofu then thawing it, makes it firm and easier to work with.
* Cooked Grains- Barley, Millet, Buckwheat, Quinoa
* Cereals- Puffed Rice, Rice Flakes, Rye Flakes, Corn Flakes, Puffed Corn, Corn Germ,
Puffed Millet, Oat Bran, Hemp, Oatmeal, Grits, Wheat-Free Granola.
* Starchy Vegetables- puree and substitute in recipes for bread, grains or pastas.

<u>SEASONINGS</u>

Salt Substitutes:
Sea Salt (NOT Iodized Salt)
Mineral Salts & Seasonings- Kelp, Sea Veggies and Herb Mixes.
Bragg's Amino Acids- great in soups and veggies (Use sparingly. Strong soy taste.)
Miso- use to taste in casseroles, gravies, sauces (a little goes a long way)
Himalayan Salt- By far, the best choice of the salts. Loaded with minerals.
Herbal Seasonings- these have very little or NO sodium
Tamari or Shoyu- use to taste in any dish needing salt. (Same as Bragg's Amino Acids)
Spices and Citrus Zest- use slightly or mixed to taste in place of salt in sweet or savory
recipes.

Sugar Substitutes:

Honey- Use ½ C. to replace sugar; reduce recipe liquid by ¼ C.
Maple Syrup (Raw/Pure)- use ½ – 2/3 C to replace 1 C sugar. reduce recipe liquid 1/4C
Molasses- use ½ C to replace 1 C sugar. Reduce recipe liquid by ¼ C.
Malt Syrup- use 1 to 1 ¼ C. to replace 1 C sugar. Reduce recipe liquid by ¼ C.

Rice Bran Syrup- (high in Silica) use same as Malt Syrup.
Apple Juice or other fruit juice- 1 C to replace 1 C sugar. Reduce recipe liquid by ¼ C.
Fructose- use 1/3 to 2/3 C to replace 1 C sugar.
Stevia Ribaudiana- sweet herb, 25 times sweeter than sugar. (Use sparingly.)
Xylitol- Made from Birch Tree sap. Slightly less sweet than sugar. Great substitute.

Note: Neither Stevia nor Xylitol will mess with your sugar. Both are great for Diabetics.

Butter substitutes:

*Vegetable Oils (cold pressed)- use in equal amounts for butter in sauces, dressings, gravies, baking and sautéing.

* Vegetable or Onion Broth- may be used instead of butter in sauces, gravies and dressings

* Clarified Butter (Ghee)- less saturated fat. To make: merely, melt butter and skim off top
foam, making sure not to disturb the melted solids. Use the clear butter in recipes as a
substitute for full-fat butter.

* Soy or Soy/Yogurt Butter- such as Brummel and Brown

* Olive Oil- use on breads as a butter substitute. (Always use Extra Virgin or Bragg's Oil)
* Olive Oil based Butter- Smart Balance, use just like butter.

HEALTHY FACTS ABOUT BUTTER

1. Butter is rich in the most easily absorb-able form of **Vitamin A** necessary for **thyroid** and **adrenal** health.
2. Contains **lauric acid**, important in treating **fungal infections** and .**candida**
3. Contains **lecithin**, essential for cholesterol metabolism.

4. Contains **anti-oxidants** that protect against **free radical damage.**
5. Has **anti-oxidants** that protect against **weakening arteries.**
6. Is a great source of **Vitamins E** and K.
7. Is a very rich source of the vital mineral **selenium.**
8. Saturated fats in butter have strong **anti-tumor** and **anti-cancer** properties.
9. Butter contains **conjugated linoleic acid**, which is a potent anti-cancer agent, muscle builder, and immunity booster
10. **Vitamin D** found in butter is essential to **absorption of calcium**.
11. Protects against **tooth decay.**
12. Is your only source of an **anti-stiffness factor,** which protects against calcification of the joints.
13. **Anti-stiffness factor** in butter also **prevents hardening of the arteries, cataracts,** and **calcification of the pineal gland**.
14. Is a source of **Activator X**, which helps your body **absorb minerals.**
15. Is a source of **iodine** in highly absorb-able form.
16. May **promote fertility** in women.
17. Is a source of quick energy and is not stored in our bodies adipose tissue.
18. Cholesterol found in butterfat is essential to **children's brain** and **nervous system** development.
19. Contains **Arachidonic Acid** (AA) which plays a role in **brain function** and is a vital component of cell membranes.
20. Protects against **gastrointestinal infections** in the very young or the elderly.

Butter from Organic, antibiotic, steroid-free animals is superior to ALL other butters.
But "over-consumption" can cause weight gain as well as numerous health issues. Use "common sense."

PEANUT BUTTER SUBSTITUTES

Place almonds, hazelnuts, pecans, walnuts, sesame seeds or
sunflower seeds in a container.
Cover with just enough water or apple juice (for sweetening)
Cover and let set overnight.
Place in food processor or blender, and mix.
Honey or applesauce may be used to sweeten.
Add a slight amount of almond or avocado oil to make pasty.
A touch of sea salt or Vega-sol may be added for spice.

Watch for:
  Dr. Mark and Sherrie's Fun and Healthy Cookbook, coming soon.

Here is a sneak preview recipe for a "Black Cow" (Root beer Float)
    1 Freeze some vanilla Almond, Rice, or Soy adding protein
powder)
                (Basically, make a vanilla protein smoothie)
    2 8 oz Perrier or Pellegrino Water +15 drops Root beer flavored
      Stevia liquid
          (or add ½ tsp Baking Soda to8 oz Distilled Water)
    3 Drop a lump of frozen smoothie in the Root beer water and
                        Voila!
                    Root beer Float.
                    And its healthy.

CHAPTER 13

PUTTING IT ALL TOGETHER

Up to this point, we have covered a lot of ground and accumulated a considerable amount of information and may have added a few complications and a little confusion to our life.

So, what do we do with all this newly found knowledge? We put it into a formula. We make it easy to understand. We make it simple.

To formulate this plan, let's make it into a health equation.

Formula for health: Diet   pH

(Y minus T + 6.4/6.4 + 80/20 + 7.4 + CS = PH)

  Y= You   T= Toxins   CS=Common PH= Perfect

                                    Sense   Health

<u>SHOPPING LIST</u>

Before we go any further, we must first go to the store and buy our supplies. Here's a shopping list of items you will need to initially get started.

For your cleanses you will need:

<u>LIVER/GALLBLADDER CLEANSE</u>
Distilled water (about 4 gallons)
Unfiltered apple juice (1-2 quarts) "Simply Apple"
Epsom's Salt
Extra Virgin Olive Oil (We suggest Bragg's)
Lemons- 4
1 quart jar w/lid

<u>INTESTINAL CLEANSE</u>
(If store bought, follow directions)
(If purchased from Castle in the Clouds) you need
Unfiltered Apple Juice (5 quarts)
<u>MASTER CLEANSE</u> (Tissues and urinary)
   (per each 2 days)

Distilled Water (1 gallon)
Lemons-8 (enough for 1 cup of juice)
Pure Maple Syrup (at least ½ cup) Spring Tree or Maple Grove

BLOOD CLEANSE TEA
Echinacea Root- 4 oz.
Burdock Root- 4 oz.
Nettle Leaves- 2 oz.
Elder Flowers, Red Clover, Peppermint- 2 oz. Each

FOODS FOR THE ALKALINE DIET

1. Lettuces: Romaine, Spinach, Green Leaf, Mixed Field Greens<
   Herb Mix, etc.
2. Vegetables: Carrots, Celery, Cucumbers, Tomatoes, Red-
   Potatoes, Zucchini, Parsley, Cilantro
3. Dairy Substitutes: Soy or Olive Oil Butter, Soy, Rice, Cashew
   or Almond Milk, Yogurt (plain and vanilla)
4. Fruit: Apples, Bananas, Blueberries, Blackberries, Figs,
Melons,
   Raspberries, Strawberries, Mangoes, Peaches, Watermelon,
   etc. You may want to get some of these frozen, for smoothies.
   You can peel and freeze bananas for this reason also.
5. Drinks: Bottled Water (or Reverse Osmosis) Herbal Teas, Fruit
Juices (not from concentrate or (juice your own) Fresh Vegetable
Juices. (The more of these the better!)
6. Fun Foods: Veggie Burgers, Veggie Dogs, Tortillas, for pizzas
7. Condiments: Bragg's Amino Acids, Bragg's Cider Vinegar,
Sea
   Salt or Himalayan Salt, Vegetable Bullion, Garlic, Balsamic-
   Vinegar.
8. Breakfast: Organic Breakfast Cereals, Organic Oatmeal,
   Organic Bread (gluten-free) Soy Bacon and Sausage.
9. Grains: Millet, Amaranth, Quinoa, Rye, Corn Meal

Now, its time to put our newly formulated health equation into a do-able format. This is the same line of protocol I place all my patients on, especially those experiencing chronic conditions

Here's a rundown of how the formula goes in action:

<u>DAY 1</u>

Liver/Gallbladder Cleanse
(no food or supplements)

<u>DAYS 2 thru 6</u>

Intestinal Cleanse
(If using Castle in the Clouds Cleanse)
small smoothies,
fresh vegetable juices
and
potassium broth
are allowed.

<u>DAY 7</u>

Master Cleanse
Lemon/Water/Maple Syrup
3 days minimum
7 days is suggested
10 days gives the ultimate results

<u>DAY 9, 13 or 16</u>
(depends on how long you did the Master Cleanse)

Breaking Your Fast

Upon Rising- 6-8 oz fresh Pineapple Juice
Wait 30 minutes- eat a piece of non-citrus fruit
Mid-Morning: 6-8 oz fresh Carrot Juice
Lunch: Vegetable Broth
Dinner: Mixed Salad w/sprouts and herbal tea
Bedtime: 1 cup Chamomile Tea

<u>DAY AFTER BREAKING FAST</u>

Time for food!

Begin the 80/20 Alkaline Eating Regime

A word of caution: Your digestive system is going to be very sensitive after having years of crude stripped away and new tissue exposed. Eat very lightly and raw for at least a week. Juice as much as possible to pre-digest the food and aid digestion.

Remember, I said,, "Listen to your body?" Now's your chance to find out what that really means. When you start to put anything in your mouth, be aware of any adverse reactions i.e., jaw rush, stomach twinge, bowel roll, a sharp pain in the jaw or stomach, any little reaction. If you get none, eat it! If so, put the food down, forever. Its not good for you.

And remember this: If you ignore these warning signs more than twice, you'll never get another subtle one until you do another cleanse. The next warning will be of the more serious kind.

Once you have finished the cleanses, you should be noticing most aches and pains, symptoms or conditions diminished greatly or disappearing completely. Arthritis pains clearing, headaches gone, fatigue replaced with vibrancy, thinking and memory improved, blood pressure, blood sugar, normalized and cholesterol improved or perfected. We have treated ourselves by cleansing the "whole" body and you now can see most of what you have been led to believe needed a doctor, has vanished.

Okay, we've emptied the room and stripped the walls and now we are ready to start painting the walls and redecorating our room.

SPECIAL BOOSTS FOR SPECIAL NEEDS

We are now ready to begin the rebuilding process. We will begin by repairing and replenishing the "Whole" body.

As you begin the 80/20 Alkaline eating Regime, if there are any remaining symptoms, this is when you will address these issues. We are continuing to treat the "Whole" body, but specific areas may require special attention or a little boost.

Arthritis- may need Raw Goat Milk, Concentrated Goat Whey (Capra Whey), Black Mission Figs as well as Glucosamine and Chondroitin with MSM and Extra EFA's (essential fatty acids). Eat and drink Alkaline

Cholesterol- (to lower) during Master Cleanse is the most effective plus 5 TBS granulated lecithin or 5 1200 IU capsules and 5 raw garlic cloves or 10 garlic caps each day for 2 weeks.

Diabetes type I and II- Pterocarpus marsupium Roxb The only known substance with the ability to re-grow pancreatic cells.

Gout- might need Black Cherry Juice and Black Mission Figs. You're too acidic

Immune System- might need an extra boost with Colostrum-1 or 2 capsules 3 x's day, L-Lysine- 1000 mg 3 x's day, 1/3 cup cottage cheese mixed with 3 TBS Flax Oil. (Eat daily for cell immunity) also Immune System Mushrooms.

I'll go over more remedies a little later on in the book.

No matter what the conditions you are faced with, this 80/20 Alkaline Regime will improve your health.

Here is what I suggest everyone takes along with this program:

Liquid Multi Vitamin/Mineral supplement
EFA's (Essential Fatty Acids) at least 2400 IU-2 x's day
Liquid Chlorophyll- 1 TBS morning and night (blood builder)
Vitamin C Powder- 5000-10000 mg daily (minimum)

LOSING WEIGHT

Here is a very popular topic. It is a craze that has men and women alike spending thousands of dollars a year on products and procedures that lead to aggravation, frustration and poor health.

As you have heard over and over and may have experienced yourself, "diets don't work." More correctly put, diets don't have a long-lasting effect. They are a short-term, temporary fix. Because they are not designed as a healthy life-style change.

Magazines and Rag-Paper diets are designed the fill pages and sell units, while TV commercial diets are designed to get quick results, get recognized and sell product.

Did you know: Americans spent over 70 billion dollars this year on dieting?

Starvation and revving up your adrenal glands with caffeine-loaded supplements are not in the best interest of the body's well-being. The toxic body also cannot naturally remove itself of unwanted fats, if its eliminative systems are blocked, hindered and not functioning properly. Remove the toxins and waste (that alone will remove weight), use the properly designed 80/20 Alkaline Eating Regime, along with the following seven basic rules of losing weight and your body will respond with a smile, steadily shrink to its ideal healthy weight, naturally sculpt itself into optimal form and put a return smile in the mirror. Best of all, you can stay this way. This is your new life-style and this is the new YOU!

Here are the rules:

1. Eat Less
2. Eat slow
3. Eat frequently
4. Chew your food well
5. Avoid <u>ALL</u> breads and dairy
6. Burn more calories than you consume
7. Move! Move! Move!

THE RULES EXPLAINED

1. **Eat less**- this is a no-brainer. You can't continue to eat the amount of food it took to keep the body at its present size. Cut your portions down and don't go for second helpings.
2. **Eat slow**- take your time eating. Slowing down the eating process gives the brain a chance to register FULL. Unless Someone is going to steal your food, no need to rush.
3. **Eat frequently**- Eating small, frequent meals keeps your metabolism going and the fat-furnace burning.
4. **Chew your food well**- Chewing our food into a liquid not only takes a load off the digestive system, but also forces you to **Rule #2**, eat slower, giving you a chance to eat less food.
5. **Avoid breads and dairy**- These are loaded with fats and calories. When consumed, they go straight to sugar, then straight to fat. Unlike the compound carbs that are almost total energy efficient.
6. **Burn more calories than you consume**- This one's pretty self-explanatory.
7. **Move**- Exercise will help support rule #6 as well as moving lymphatic fluids, helping to further remove toxins, tone your body, strengthen your muscles, keep you supple and work your cardiovascular system. Besides, why not start sculpting, so when all that good stuff is exposed, it'll already be lookin' good!

These exercises should be included in some form:

    a. Cardio- Walking , jogging, aerobics, Rebounder, Tai-Bo, Tai Chi, Biking, etc.

    b. Stretching- Slow, easy stretching pre-workout, prevents injury as well as keeping the muscles limber. Yoga is wonderful for this.

    c. Weight lifting- Strengthens muscles and bones and tones. No need to lift heavy weights unless you are trying to bulk up.

    d. Breathing- Deep breathing exercises help remove stale air from the lungs and brings much needed oxygen to the cellular level and calms the mind and spirit. Good to do each morning and after exercise. Yoga Tantric Breathing is a controlled method, great for clearing the sinus, expanding the lung, clearing the air and bringing massive amounts of oxygen in.

One of my favorite ways of oxygenating is singing. If singing is not your passion or you are asked to find a new method of oxygenation, try "hissing." Simply take a deep breath, in through your nose, and slowly "hiss" the air out through your teeth. Try longer periods of hissing with each breath. Try one stop-light to another. Its fun, you are bettering your health as you drive, and people will think you're crazy when they drive up beside you with your teeth clenched and lips pursed like an angry tiger and your face is tinted a strange, but beautiful shade of ozone blue.

CHAPTER 14

YOUR ALTERNATIVE PHARMACY

Angina Medication: L- Theanine (anxiety)
> Hawthorn Berry, tea, tincture or caps
> L-Carnitine

Anti-acids: Baking Soda

Arthritis- Glucosamine/Chondroiton, MSM
> Water, more water

Asthma and Antihistamines-
> Water in high quantities

Blood Pressure Lowering-
> Nattokinase
> Water and plenty of it.

Cholesterol Lowering-
> Garlic-10 caps or 5 raw cloves a day
> Lecithin-10 caps or 5 TBS granules a day
> Niacin- 100 mg 3x's day
> Gugulipid- 25 mg 3x's day
> Omega 3/6/9 Fatty Acids- 2400 IU day
> Pectin- 20 grams a day. Eat 2-3 servings fruit
> a day
> Reduce or omit animal meats and biproducts.
> Stop the source.

Cold Medications-
> Vitamin C 2,000 – 3,000 mg every 4 hours
> Echinacea- 1 gram 3x's day (tea or capsules)
> Golden Seal- 1,000-2000 mg 3x's day (Take
> for no more than 2 weeks.)
> Omni-Immune- 6 drops 2x's day
> Zinc Lozenges- 1 every 2 hours for 1 week
> Baking Soda ¼- ½ tsp in juice, 3x's day
> Drink plenty of water
> Cold Remedy Tea- Juice a 1 inch Ginger
> slice, 1 raw garlic clove and the juice
> of ½ lemon. Add to warm or cool
> apple juice. Dose: 3 cups per day.

Corticosteroids-

   Pancreatin 500-1000 mg 3x's day
   Bromelain 400-600 mg a day for inflammation.
   Wobenzymes- 3-6 capsules, 3x's day
   Vital-zymes- 3-6 capsules 3x's day
   Curcumin- 400-600 micrograms 3x's day

Diabetes Medications-

   Chromium 200-400 micrograms daily
   Manganese- 30 mg daily
   Zinc- 30 mg daily
   Biotin- 20 mg daily
   Colostrum- 2 caps or 1 tsp powder 3 a day
   Omni-Immune-6-15 drops once a day
   Eat high fiber and low sugar diet
   Drink lots of water

Headache Med-

   Migraines-Magnesium Aspartate 500 mg day
   Feverfew capsules 25 mg caps 2x's day
   (and 1-2 grams to combat acute attack)
   Check for food allergies
   Common Headache- White Willow Bark

Laxatives-

   Cascara Sagrada and Senna in capsules 2-4
   morning and evening for 1 week maximum.
   Epsoms Salt- 1-2 Tbs in 1 qt. distilled water
   Bladderwack- relaxes colon. 2-3 caps 2x's day
   Frangula Bark- restore toning to the large
   intestine
   Drink plenty of water
   Eat high fiber and bulk

Prostate-

   Saw palmetto- 4 mg 3x's day
   Zinc- 50-100 mg day (no more)
   Pumpkin Seeds
   Sesame Seeds

Thyroid-

   Hyper or Hypo- Iodine 12.5 mg 1-3x's day
   Thyroid-S from Thailand
  (No thyroid meds will work unless iodine level is up)

Sedative Medication-

  Magnesium 400-800 mg before bed
  Melatonin-must be 10 mg
  Valerian Root-tea or tincture

Weight Loss Med.- |

  Read detoxing and weight loss chapters.

CHAPTER 15

HOW HEALTHY DO YOU WANT TO GET?

Now that you're seeing how the body accumulates toxins, sludge and debris in various ways from how we eat to environmental elements. (mostly from the way we eat) You see how important it is to put the proper nutrients into the body using the finest ingredients possible. You see that if we don't become aware and take actions of prevention, we are slowly causing disease, digging our own grave and cutting our life short.

If you are experiencing health problems, want to prevent health problems in the future, or just want to regain and retain your health and vitality, do your cleanses first. "Always do your cleanses first." Its our own choice just how healthy we want to become or not become.

We've discussed Vegetarianism vs the Carnivore diet and in most cases, the "Scavenger" diet. Again, vegetarianism is NOT for everyone. However, done correctly, it is the ultimate choice in regaining and maintaining optimal health and prolonging longevity.

Don't want to get quite that radical? Then, may I suggest, as I had stated before, eliminate beef and pork completely out of your diet. Eat fish, chicken, turkey and wild game, all baked, broiled or grilled and ALL organic.

Never fry ANYTHING. Of course, with wild game, you hope they haven't been grazing on pesticide-ladened land.

Stay away from ALL foods with preservatives, food coloring, hydrogenated oils, table salt, caffeine, bleached white flour, processed sugar, gluten and GMO'd foods. I know I've said all this several times before and I'll probably say it again, before its all over. I want you to get it.

Take a good Liquid Multi Vitamin/Mineral supplement. We suggest Intra-Max vitamins. They are made from live foods, all organic, contain 415 nutrients and we feel they are unsurpassed in quality and effectiveness. 100% Instantly absorbed into your bloodstream.

Okay, after hearing all this information on eating for optimal health, you may say, "That's still a bit too radical for me. I like beef, I like my occasional pizza with all the gooey cheese and mushrooms and pepperoni. After a hot summer day, I like to eat my ice-cream. I don't like vegetables. I want my cereal. I want my eggs and bacon for breakfast and maybe a side of biscuits and sausage gravy. I like to eat! I don't want to change my eating habits." All I can say to you is…Good Luck!

You may think your body is capable of taking this abuse, but beware. The body will reach its level of tolerance and when it does, every bit of that junk-ladened food is going to come crashing down on you like an avalanche.

But, I'm not going to give up on you yet. You could still consume most of these favorite foods and still not place yourself in an early grave. You could eat less meat but make it organic. Make your own pizza using healthy ingredients. Make baked fries instead of greasy fries or get an airless fryer. (They are cool!) Try making a smoothie and freezing it for ice-cream, they're awesome. You can substitute all the bad foods you like to eat with healthy-cooked versions. Find out how in the "Food Substitution" section.

I'm STILL not giving up on you, yet. If you just don't want to give up those old eating habits, at least do the cleanses or at least some of the cleanses, a Liver/Gallbladder and Colon cleanse. You will be giving your liver and colon some room to breathe. You will, for the time being anyway, hold off the doctors, medications and operations you are destined to be facing otherwise.

Now, if you won't even try a cleanse to help yourself, I give up. If I care more about your health than you do about your own health, your spirit may be in the grave already. It's time you do some inner searching and learn how important you are. Learn to love that person inside. Learn to feel good about that person looking back at you every morning in the mirror.

JUST DO IT!

(THE POWER SECTION)

If you're still with me, you should be revved up and ready to do some changing. I'm the kind of person who likes to challenge the challenge. My belief is, "If you want it done, DO IT!" This

209

chapter is dedicated to those of you who want to "do it."
This is Dr. Mark's "don't beat around the bush" methodology,
better known as:

"Dr. Mark-o-dology."

* If you're fat and **want to lose weight**, stop eating fat, eat less
and burn more calories than you shove in. DO IT!

*If you have **High Cholesterol**, lower your consumption of or
stop eating anima products altogether. That's where it ALL
comes from. DO IT!

* If you have **High Blood Pressure**, detox and go on raw foods
for a month, cut out the salt, cut out the fat, cut out the cigarettes
and alcohol and keep calm. DO IT!

* If you have **Diabetes**, lose weight, detox, stop consuming
sugar, eat more fiber and drink more water. DO IT!

* If you have **sinus problems, allergies** or **asthma**, stop eating
dairy, wheat and gluten. Drink more water. DO IT!

* If you have **arthritis**, do the Master Cleanse, eat raw, drink
goat whey, eat black mission figs and get alkaline. DO IT!

* If you have **gout**, do a full body detox, stop eating acidic meat
and drinking acidic alcohol, Use black cherry juice, take Baking
Soda baths, get alkaline and DO IT! (1 box Baking Soda in hot
bath. Soak 20 minutes)

* If you're **tired**, you're probably toxic. Do ALL the cleanses
and eat alkaline, electricity-producing foods)

* If you have **bowel** and **digestive problems**, do the cleanses and
eat sensibly. Follow the 80/20 diet.

* If you're suffering from **depression**, clean the colon, clean the
blood, clean your mind and meditate. Eat Alkaline. DO IT!

* If you suffer from **impotency**, clean out ALL the systems, stop ALL fried foods and grease, sodas and caffeine, take 3,000 to 6,000 mg of L-Arginine a day and Make Love! DO IT!

* If you're **irritable** and **angry**, clean out your colon, clean out your mind and possibly take a closer look at the image in the mirror. DO IT!

* If you suffer from **chronic fatigue** or **fibromyalgia**, do ALL the cleanses, change your diet to 80/20 alkaline, change your mind, alkalize and let go of the disease. DO IT!

* If you have **weak, puny muscles**, exercise. Eat some whey-protein, amino acids, break down those muscle fibers and build new ones. DO IT!

* If you want to **stop smoking**, the best time is during the cleanses. The toxins are flushed out faster than they can react.
DO IT!

* If you want to end **alcohol** or **drug addiction**, do the cleanses, take a deep breathe, smile and enjoy your new life.   DO IT!

* If you have **cancer**, do ALL the cleanses, stop ALL processed sugar consumption, go on the 80/20 regime, avoid ALL meats, breathe slow and deeply, develop a healing mental attitude and stay positive. DO IT!

* If you suffer from **osteoporosis**, do ALL the cleanses, alkalize your body and replace the missing calcium and magnesium with good organic sources. DO IT!

Returning the body to a perfect state of health is different for each individual. Some will see instant results, while others may take a little longer.

*"Your body heals itself from the inside out
and from top to bottom, in that order."*

This is known as "Herring's Law.

This is the law of Mother Nature. Nature knows what its doing and the time it needs to take to do it. The deepest set in illness(s) will be the first to go. The <u>line of most resistance</u> will be the one to get the first attention. *"Squeaky wheel gets the grease!"*

Keep at it, don't give up, don't get discouraged and don't quit.

Mother Nature will do what she needs to do, as she needs to do it. Don't force her or she'll push back. Don't complain to her because the second half of that old adage is:

"and the noisy crow…gets shot!"

Trust her, she is a kind and gentle soul. Love her, for she'll never do her children wrong.

JUST SOME FUN STUFF

1. White blood cells live about 2 days, red blood cells about 4 months. In 3-4 months, your whole blood supply is replaced. Brain cells can live over 60 years.
2. In six months, almost all the proteins in your body are replaced, even the DNA in your genes.
3. In one year, all the bones and even the enamel on your teeth are replaced, constructed entirely of the nutrients you eat.
4. A human being needs a daily intake of: 60 minerals, 16 vitamins, 8 essential amino acids and 3 essential fatty acids.
5. All disease is caused by a mineral deficiency, toxins or both.
6. "Death" is the body's "end saturation" of acid.
7. Proper urine and saliva pH's are 6.4 pH respectively.
8. Perfect body tissue pH is 7.4 pH, making it disease resistant.
9. Colloidal minerals are too large for proper and complete assimilation. Angstrom-sized particles are 10,000 times smaller than a colloid.
10. Graying hair is a sign of "copper" deficiency.
11. Coral calcium will NOT build one single cell of bone. It is also NOT made from "living coral" as living coral reefs are protected by law. Coral calcium is merely limestone deposits left from coral reefs that are now dead. Calcium must be of the "hydroxide" type, to build bone.

12. Osteoporosis, is caused from an over-acidic constitution. Calcium is the body's natural acid-buffer. The bones are the closet and most plentiful source of this calcium. When the buffering calcium is removed, we are left with voids. Magnesium stops osteoporosis dead in its tracks!
13. Multiple Sclerosis is caused by "Leaky Gut" syndrome. These are perforations made in the intestinal walls by the over-use of pain killers, prescription drugs, aspirin, alcohol, sodas, and highly acid-forming foods.
14. Vitamin C, is the cement that holds all of our cells together. As we deplete our supply, we begin to wrinkle.
15. Vitamin C, MUST be present for the formation of collagen.
16. Humans cannot manufacture or produce Vitamin C internally. All of the ingredients are present in our DNA but the recipe has not been written.
17. Goats produce approximately 13,000 mg of Vitamin C daily. If put under stress, a goat may produce upwards of 40,000 milligrams a day.
18. Guinea pigs cannot produce Vitamin C. That is why they are used in laboratories. You cannot stress-induce an illness that is capable of producing vitamin C.
19. All wild animal produce vitamin C. This is why the majority live disease-free until death.
20. Domesticated dogs and cats produce about 10% of the vitamin C that wild animals produce. This is why they fall prey to illness before they die.
21. One "cure" for arthritis is to take some KFC chicken, throw away the skin and the meat, cook the ends of the bones, then pulverize them with a hammer and take 2 ½ ounces a day. However, it is said, you may get thrown in jail because you will be practicing medicine?
22. Your liver has over 1000 functions to perform. Next to your brain, it is the most important organ in your body.
23. During your lifetime, your liver will supply over 6 billion different types of enzymes. During a day, your liver will produce 4 to 5 billion enzymes in quantity.
24. You have 1/6 oz or 3.25 grams of iron in your body. That's about enough to make a "10 penny" nail.
25. 100 trillion atoms make up one cell.

You have 75 trillion cells in your body.
99.9999% of every atom is empty space.
What does that make us….an illusion?
26. Potassium Iodide will eliminate fibroid tumors.

CHAPTER 16

QUICK RE-CAP FOR PERFECT HEALTH

1. Your blood is only as clean as your colon.
2. Clean blood means a healthy body.
3. You do not live off the food you eat, but off the electricity produced by the digestion of that food.
4. Eat for electricity. Eat live foods with enzymes still intact.
5. Keep body tissue at 7.4 pH and disease resistant with 80/20 alkaline food regime.
6. Eat 60% of your vegetables raw and 40% cooked.
7. For maximum potential energy, keep urine and saliva pH's at 6.4 pH, monitoring with litmus paper or pH meter.
8. Avoid greasy, fried foods, trans-fats and hydrogenated oils.
9. Avoid ALL preservatives except for vitamin E (tocopherols) and vitamin C.
10. Avoid ALL foods containing food coloring. Read your labels.
11. Avoid processed sugars.
12. Stay away from caffeine and stimulants (sodas, coffee, caffeine teas, alcohol, etc.)
13. Reduce or totally avoid dairy (milk, cheese, ice-cream, etc.)
14. Avoid red meat and pork
15. All other meats should be baked, broiled or grilled.
16. Do ALL cleanses every 6 months for optimal health.
17. Drink half your body weight in ounces of water.
18. Exercise daily. 10-30 minutes.
19. Never cook with aluminum cook-wear.
20. Keep a clear and positive mind. Meditate daily.
21. Breathe deep. Breathe slow. Oxygenate those cells.
22. Keep clean, think clean and you will restore and maintain absolute health and your youthfulness.
23. Eat slow and chew your food.

THINK THAT AND THAT YOU SHALL BECOME

"Your reality is what YOU believe in!"

We've all heard the old adage, "You are what you eat." If we eat high electricity foods and take the proper supplements that contain or replenish the needed or missing frequencies, we will sustain a healthy status to our physical body.

Health is: "the state of energy your body is in.
"If an organ is slacking, the proper frequency is lacking."
I did not intend for that to rhyme, but it did. If we have a darkened area in our "aura," our light bulb, our electro-magnetic field, (the harmonious sum of our total electrical output) there is a missing electrical frequency(s) in the meridian attached to that specific area. (Meridians, being specific pathways in the human body where within, energy flows from one point to another.) Replenish that frequency(s) with the proper one, through means of food, supplements, color therapy, bio-electrical device or controlled thought, and that darkened are is restored to the vibrance of the rest of the auric output.

Let's take this "healthy physical energy" concept one step further. Our whole universe is set up on the "Energy Follows Intent" principle. Meaning, that when energy (or a thought in this case) is manifested, it begins to materialize or "snowball" from that point forward until it meets its end point, which would be its coming into existence.

Now, just for the fun of it, let's write and direct our own sci-fi movie. We have to have a name for our movie, so let's call it, "The Snowball of My Life." We have a whole great big empty screen to fill up with anything we want to fill it with. We only have one rule, "We always have two choices." That's it!

Now, let's set the scene:

Okay, here we are, standing on top of a hill with all the power of the Universe. One side of the hill is very steep, with many objects and obstacles all the way down. It also points towards a very largely populated city.

The other side of the hill is more gradual, more gently sloped and less cluttered. It's a little less exciting and leads towards an ugly, unpopulated, dried up desert. (Sounds like we're standing atop Calico Basin in Las Vegas where I used to meditate.) Remember, we always have two choices.

Now, let's make a very small snowball, no bigger than a thought, and let's initially and intently choose to aim our snowball down the more populated side of the hill. After all, this could lead to quite an exciting scene for our movie with all those unsuspecting people down there.

Here we go, "and…action!"

With cameras rolling, we give a push and our little snowball is on its way. Unobstructed, it continues rolling the hill, faster and faster, so fast the cameraman can barely keep up.

Gathering more size, more speed and more momentum, growing larger and larger with every rotation, our little snowball begins to resemble a small planet, devouring everything in its path, (there went the cameraman) becoming the largest and most devastating snowball in the history of giant snowballs rolling down a hill, so large and out-of-control that Bruce Willis and Will Smith put together couldn't stop it!

And just as all things must come to an end, our planet-sized snowball rolls into the center of a huge city, (Shoot, let's make this movie really exciting and instead of a city, let's make it "Planet Earth!) smashing and destroying everything in sight, leaving nothing but a giant pile of wreckage where the Earth once used to be. All of our budget, our precious time and our footage was lost with the cameraman. Next, we discover, even if we had finished the movie, everyone that would have come to see it was extinguished in the crash!

However, being the director of this movie, we have another option, remember, we have another option, our second choice. Luckily, we can opt for and create an alternative ending.

This time, in the initial beginning, just to see what happens, let's aim our thought-sized snowball 180 degrees in the other direction, down the less steeper and less cluttered side of the hill.

And…action!

And just like our first snowball, it begins rolling down the other side of the hill, growing larger and getting faster. But this time, instead of knocking down trees and destroying anything and everything there is to destroy, it begins gathering seeds and all the beautiful grasses and flowers of all kinds, until it gently and peacefully comes to rest in an ugly, dried up, desolate desert, begins to melt and run, distributing the seeds and all the beautiful grasses and wildflowers it had accumulated along its path, turning this once, dried up, ugly desert into a beautiful utopia, bursting with all the colors of Springtime and creating a brand new, beautiful world that had never existed before.

"And…cut!"

Yes, thoughts are very powerful indeed. They can heal or they can destroy. One thought can infect an entire planet.

A thought is comprised of energy molecules. Your cells operate on these electrical frequencies as impulses. The right frequency makes the cell feel good and operate optimally. The wrong frequency makes the cell sick and unable to perform in an adequate manner or not at all.

Did you know: Every thought that's produced in your brain, reverberates down through every single cell in your body before it goes out into the rest of the world? They are also comprised of pure energy. Now, we know, energy can't bee destroyed. So, guess what?... Snowballs!

This is a powerful thing and one of the magic keys to good health. Every thought you think is filtered down through every one of the 75 trillion cells that make up your body. (Similar to having mud on your shoes and tracking across the kitchen floor. We all know how much trouble that can cause.) We are now beginning to see how we mentally control our health, our world and our very destiny from our own thought process.

If we produce mean, angry thoughts, we inject negative energy into each of our cells. Likewise, if we produce loving, healthy, happy thoughts, we are nurturing our cells and providing them with positive, healthy, stimulating energy.

A physical cell runs on energy, so such, for everything that exists and operates on the spiritual plane. Your spirit is energy, as well. Now, we all know body, mind and spirit must work in harmony with one another. So, total health and well-being is just that… having body, mind and spirit working harmoniously or having a perfectly balanced sum of energy. The perfect "aura."

This is not just a New Age, Ram Das, guru, philosophical statement. This is being scientifically proven through quantum physics.

Thought IS a powerful tool. Thought is energy and it can govern whether a person is healthy or not or recovers from a serious ailment or not.

Energy is universal. Like fish in an ocean all being connected by the water in the ocean, all that exists in the Universe is connected through energy. The energy of the universe is constantly flowing into your body and back out again. If your brain conjures a negative thought, that thought is reverberated down through your body, diseasing every cell in your body.

As this universal flow passes through your cells, now infected with your negative thought energy, it exists your body, and returning to the universe, slowly infects all.

You, as only one person's thoughts, may seem trivial in this huge universe. It would take a long time to fill a swimming pool up with water one drop at a time, but it would eventually happen. Think if many people were to join you and add their drops.

Likewise, "positive" energy has the ability to "heal," Infect yourself with positive thought and heal yourself. Them, infect…
the Universe!

The power of the mind is unlimited and always present. The belief in the power of the mind is fragile. One must know his or her limitations and one will soon find out, there are none.

The searcher who crosses the veil of disbelief crosses into the infinite, limitless powers of the Universe. He will find that link, which links each to one another, every cell, every molecule and every particle of matter in existence. That link is <u>energy</u>. You are energy. The Universe is energy. Every particle of matter in the universe is connected to every other particle of matter throughout the universe by way of energy. Just as all the fishes in the sea are connected by the very water they live in, we too are connected to everything existing in the universe, by the ocean of energy in which we live. This means, even though unaware of the fact, we are connected to particles, cells and molecules light-years and galaxies away. This is very exciting. We are connected to ALL there is. This makes us "Omni-Present."

IN CLOSING

 Dear Friends,

Energy cannot be destroyed. We can split atoms, smash quarks but we can never, never destroy energy. This is truly awesome because all thought is comprised of pure energy, and if energy is everlasting, that means every thought that has ever been projected since the beginning of consciousness, is floating somewhere out in Cyberspace, just waiting to be harnessed, waiting to become an "intent," waiting to be reborn and re-instated into conscious existence.

Energy can never die. It may change forms, but it can never die. It is "omni-present," constantly flowing in and out of your being for as long as you remain a being. This energy flows in and this energy flows out, making you a part of that energy. You are made up of this energy. This is the energy or electricity that gives you the title of a "living being." That makes you one with the whole universe. That <u>makes</u> <u>you</u> the universe. And if you are the universe, why can you not make anything happen you desire or "intend"? Take control.

Try it. No matter what your illness and no matter what the odds, no matter what modality you choose to endeavor, say, "I am beating this thing!" And guess what? You already have. It's not magic, its not voodoo, it's simply the way the universe is set up. A very wise soul once stated, "You shall do as great and greater things than I." What does that tell you? Its yours! The Universe and all its power, is yours for the using. Use it wisely. Use it for all your needs. Use it for the needs of others. Use it to heal yourself. Use it to heal the world. But use it wisely. Use it for positive growth. When you learn you can have anything you want just by believing and knowing it <u>will</u> come to be, you <u>will</u> heal yourself and heal your life. You will have become "One with the Universe" or "One with the Force," Luke Skywalker. Decide how you want to use it, "ask, and ye shall receive."

Don't just read this stuff, use it ! Its ALL just part of the goodies in the back-pack you were issued, when you became a human-being. Think well and then stay that way!

This is your life's story,
                  write it anyway you want.

If you want to live to be one hundred fifty….
why not?

This has been a fun ride. Thanks for sharing it with me.

Until we meet again,
Dr. Mark

Read: Dr. Mark Sexton's "The Human Repair Manual" for even more information on keeping your body healthy and running far beyond its warranty limitations.

Some more fun Did you knows:

Did you know: Statin drugs suppress your liver's ability to make cholesterol? It actually processes it from fat and guess what, not only is it LDL but its actually VLDL (very low density lipo-protein)

Did you know: Your liver uses cholesterol to flush itself out?

Did you know: Your liver sends the cholesterol to the glands for making cholesterol-based hormones like estrogen, testosterone and progesterone?

Did you know: Your brain by weight is 50% cholesterol?

Did you know: Your nervous system uses massive amounts LDL cholesterol?

Did you know: Your cholesterol-based hormones are made from LDL the "BAD" cholesterol? As well as the brain? As well as all your vessels in the circulatory system?

Did you know: It is now been estimated that 80% of Alzheimer's Disease is caused from "statin" drugs?

Did you know: By suppressing the liver with statin drugs, you're turning off its ability to clean itself, to make hormone bases, to feed the brain, to nourish the central nervous system?

Did you know: By taking these drugs you are setting yourself up for hormonal imbalances, liver damage, neuro-logical imbalances and dementia, Brain disease or Alzheimer's Disease?

Did you know: High LDL doesn't cause strokes or heart disease.

Did you know: Your nerves are 50% cholesterol?

Did you know: 1 packet of Nutra-Sweet destroys 50% gut flora?

Did you know: 80% of ALL the antibiotics produced in the US
go into animal meat?
Did you know: Pain killers, such as Morphine, not only put the |
pain receptors to sleep, but the immune system,
digestive, respiratory and ALL other systems and
body functions including your brain and even legs?

My last pieces of advice: If its been labeled "incurable" or "genetics," it is almost ALWAYS caused from toxins and in most cases, can be COMPLETELY eradicated. It just takes: cleansing, determination and persistence. From simply doing the cleanses, I have witnessed the eradication of, COPD, diabetes, HBP, allergies, Autism, Lupus, MS, Arthritis, Seizures, Infertility, skin disorders, Hemochromatosis, Polycythemia Vera and many so called "untreatable" conditions.

Cell Phones and 5G

Always keep a cell phone 2-3 inches away from your head or use your speaker phone. If Blue Tooth is going through your headset, ear buds, etc. it WILL cause a brain tumor. The only safe headsets are the hollow tubes type. Wires will conduct radiation. **right** to your brain. DO NOT carry cell phones in your pocket or purse. They WILL cause cancer. 5G emits 10x's more radiation than 4G.

The powers that be, would like you to think these waves are harmless. They have rushed this new technology onto the market without any testing to determine the health risks associated with 5G. It has already been proven that 4G causes brain tumors and organ cancers. The first symptom is a cataract developing on the same side of your face use most use your cell phone. 5G is 10 times more powerful.

Many persons have developed Radio Frequency Sensitivity Disease meaning, they become severely reactive when exposed to radio frequencies. Many suffer internal bleeding which eventually leads to stomach cancer. I have had several male patients with testicular cancer from a cell phone being carried in the pocket. Yes, they each lost a testicle.

Children are most susceptible up to 12 years of age, as the cell phone radiation, due to very thin skull bones, penetrates completely through the brain.

Mylar pouches may be purchased for carrying your phone. These repel the RF from reaching your body. This is the material potato chip bags are made. Yes, doubling up a chip bag and placing it around the phone will act as a make-shift shield.

5G technology will be fast, some awesome, but deadly.
Keep your cell phones away from your bodies at ALL times.

In a Nutshell

Three easy steps for eradicated 90% of ALL illnesses:
1. Complete Body Detox
2. Eat the Alkaline Diet
3. 90 essential nutrients for repair and maintenance
   That's it, plain and simple.

Simple Explanation

1. Removes toxins and disruptive electrical frequencies
2. Immunes your body to disease and maintains frequencies.
3. Provides ALL building blocks for remaining healthy.

Bottom line, this is ALL you need to know.

If this does not completely eradicate your condition, you can make an appointment with Doctor Mark for a private phone consultation to discuss the remaining symptoms and possible solutions.

Take charge of your health…

Take back your life…

and

LIVE!

Appendix

Product	Purchase from
Intestinal Cleansing Package	Castle in the Clouds L.L.C.
D-Oxygenator	Castle in the Clouds L.L.C.
GB-4000 Rife Machine	Castle in the Clouds L.L.C.
Omni-Immune	Castle in the Clouds L.L.C.
Intra-Max Liq. Vitamin/Minerals	Castle in the Clouds L.L.C.
Black Salve	Castle in the Clouds L.L.C.

All above products may be ordered directly from:
www.castlesexton@hotmail.com   or call: 573-317-1912

Thyroid-S	www.thyroidthailand.com
LDN (Low dose Naltrexone)	www.buylowdosenaltrexone.com
Ultra-Liquid Zeolite w/DHQ	http://zeolite.com
Color Therapy Kit	www.productsondemand.biz

Products on Demand
1-203-322-1774

For color therapy I suggest these items:
   Par-can Light
  "Let There Be Light"- book
   Roscolene Filter set (I prefer the complete filter kit)
   Variant Breath Calendar

ORDERING INFORMATION

**All products mentioned in this book, if not listed above, may be
purchased directly from Castle in the Clouds' store-front at:**

www.DSSOrders.com/CastleInTheCloudsLLC
Use this special code: **MS2091**

More books from Dr. Mark Sexton:

  "I'll Miss You in the Moon" -Sherrie/Mark Sexton
  "Romantic Poetry for the Soul"- Mark Sexton
  "The Human Repair Manual"- Dr. Mark Sexton N.D. PhD

The D-OXY oxygen bath overview

For many years, world renowned Castle in the Clouds L.L.C. has been using this technology exclusively as a service to their patients with some very amazing effects. The original machine cost upwards of $30,000.00. After many requests and twenty years of experimentation and re-design we were able to bring this once out-of-reach technology down to a price the general public can afford.

The D-OXY or (Destabilized Oxygen) machine does just what the name implies. The hydrogen molecules are released from the oxygen molecule bond, creating a very un-stabilized oxygen environment, wherein "Atomic Oxygen" or multiple oxygen molecules are linked creating bonds of what used to be singlet oxygen molecules, to new groups of super oxygenated bonds of 30 or more oxygen molecules. Oxygen can sustain this massive instability for only brief moments in time and begin cascading downward to search for a more stable state of being. However, in the interim of this hyper-saturated, cascading event, the very vulnerable toxins, free radicals and pathogens are destroyed by this super powerful oxygen form.

The oxygen is up taken trans-dermally, meaning, through the skin, therefore, there is no danger of hyper-saturation of carbon dioxide or circulatory damage due to excessive oxygen delivery such as with a hyperbolic or hyperbaric chamber. There is also no limitation to the time one may remain or how often one may partake in one of the D-OXY oxygen machines. Many laboratory tests have proven this oxygen machine to be far superior in oxygen delivery as well as patient recovery time and applicational safety.

The D-OXY machine does not make oxygen. It is unique in that it is separating the oxygen molecules from the hydrogen molecules, causing the non-stabilized oxygen molecules to group up and become basically electroplated into groups, creating long chain oxygen molecules, much resembling long chain amino acids. Hence, instead of the typical singlet oxygen molecule being used up and expelled in the normal fifteen seconds or less as seen with the breathing in of oxygen, the long chain oxygen molecules are absorbed through the skin and stay fully intact and activated for six to eight hours, giving a very much extended working period than the usual fifteen seconds. A person or patient can be kept totally saturated with the powerful healing effects of oxygen 24/7. This means tremendous recovery potential in a much shorter period of time than the typical oxygen delivery systems. A second natural and very beneficial effect occurs as the "O" molecules are stripped from the hydrogen. This separation leaves the hydrogen in a paired molecular state hence becoming one of the strongest anti-oxidants known to the scientific community.

This two-fold alteration makes for a very powerful healing modality that will super-saturate the entire interior and exterior of the body. Every cell is pumped to maximum oxygen capacity, as well as every interstitial space between the cells. The result is a massive detoxification through oxidation, as well as the removal and destruction of many unfavorable pathogens such as viruses, fungi, yeast and bacteria.

It has recently been discovered, the D-OXY machine is producing 4th Phase water, the state of water inside each and every cell of the human body, crucial to your health and life itself, has been pointed out as another reason for the almost immediate healing results observed and experienced using the D-Oxy bath.

The D-OXY machine is not just for the sick. Athletes also find favorable results by greatly-enhanced athletic performances, increased endurance and maximum sustainability to quicker recovery time from injuries as well. The D-OXY is not just for athletes either. Every human as well as animals will find great benefits from taking a one-hour D-OXY bath. Greater clarity of mind, more energy, greater awareness, clearer skin, enhanced immunity from illnesses and much more have been experienced by many. Animal injuries and skin conditions have been improved as well.

Wonderful results have been witnessed by many persons with a wide variety of ailments and conditions. Skin rashes, greatly improved or eliminated in a short period of time. Stroke victims benefit from the increased oxygen to the brain. Respiratory ailments such as emphysema and COPD quickly find an increase in breathing ease and capacity. Many have been able to function without further need of medications. Fungi, such as Candida are generally eradicated or brought in check in a short one-hour bath time. Cuts and serious open wounds are aided in their closing by the powerful supersaturation of these long-chain oxygen molecules. Many have seen extreme cases of varicose veins completely disappear, avoiding costly and sometimes painful removal procedures.

Oxygen is the healer of healers and there is no other method on the market that can deliver this powerful and crucial element into the human body. The D-OXY is compact, lightweight and very portable. It is self-contained complete with a self-priming pump. It needs simply plugged in to a 110v AC outlet, the two hoses placed in a bathtub or spa tub full of water and turned on. There is a brief 15 to 20-minute oxygen saturation charging of the water that needs to take place and it is ready to go.

The D-Oxygenator is lightweight, very portable and can be plumbed directly into a bathtub or hot-tub.

Each machine is produced as ordered and fully tested before leaving our facility.

More information is available upon request.

www.castlesexton@hotmail.com

or

573-317-1912

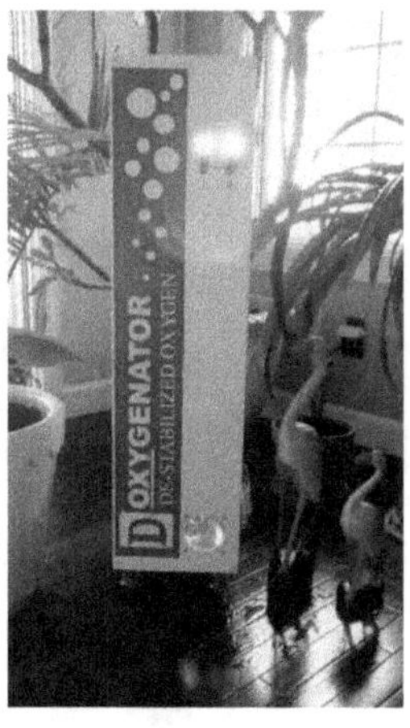

"D-Oxygenator"

www.ingramcontent.com/pod-product-compliance
Lightning Source LLC
Chambersburg PA
CBHW061753250726
48657CB00001B/99